"*Run Yourself Happy* is a wonderful resource for anyone who desires to harness the full potential of mind, body and spirit through the activity of running."

Lisa Engles,
Author of *Breathe Run Breathe*,
Creator of the Breathe Run Breathe Running Program,
Head Running Coach, Silicon Valley Triathlon

"As a former high school and collegiate runner I enjoy Carrie's fresh outlook on how to make running fun again. I utilize these techniques personally, and also share with the high school athletes I now coach."

Kareen Nilsson Shackelford
NCAA All American
Cross Country and Track Coach

Praise for *Run Yourself Happy*

"Carrie Roldan has created a unique, energized and powerful method to gain happiness and fulfillment into your life, tune into who you are, and add peace to your life. This book motivates the reader to move, meditate and manifest. Her authenticity and down to earth attitude draw the reader in to relate and be inspired.

Kim Somers Egelsee
#1 bestselling author of *Getting Your Life to a Ten +*

"*Run Yourself Happy* is a wonderfully written book that begins with a very personal, inspiring story of a woman who has found herself in a very dark place. Through laughter, love, service, and running she is able to turn her life around and find her true calling. Carrie Roldan's genuine and personal style gives the reader a wonderful sense of companionship and honesty. As you continue to read, you witness how powerful each of us really are. You learn by simply going for a run you too can find true happiness.

"After reading *Run Yourself Happy*, I have developed two 'mantras' I want to live my life by- to do what inspires me, and to live with love.

"I love this book because it is written to affect you differently at different times in your life. You can use its masterful concepts to *stay* happy. This book has the ability to change your entire concept of what happiness is, and what living happy is all about. So be ready, say your goodbyes to anxiety, depression, and hate, and take this book and *run* with it!"

Mike Chavez, PT
Owner at Stride Ahead Coaching

"I am so excited about Carrie Roldan's leading edge book, *Run Yourself Happy*. Carrie brings her intuitive, heartful, and inspiring approach, and engages the commitment of her readers to 'decide to be happy' and discover the joys of running as meditation in action. Carrie brings ease and integrity to the science of running, and combines them with her understandings from the spiritual and happiness realms. Clearly, a life-changing tool and process, this book is sure to empower many."

Laura Jane,
Author of *Simple Everyday Prenatal Radiance*

"Regular runners intuitively understand that running is much more than just running and so *Run Yourself Happy* is a must read for every runner. But, it is the impact this book could have in a world where inactivity has become the norm that excites me the most. *Run Yourself Happy* provides some powerful reasons for people to get outdoors and exercise, especially those who have yet to find the joys of living in peace and purpose in their daily lives.

Jim Kirwan
Founder of Get America Moving ™

"This book is a must read for runners and yogis alike. Carrie Roldan integrates so many soulful practices into running that will evoke and inspire a sense of divine connection, personal awareness, and encourage you to allow yourself to feel the joy that is always within."

Denise Dare
Happiness Artist/Blogger/ Life Coach

Run Yourself Happy

A FIVE WEEK TRAINING PROGRAM TO RELEASE ANXIETY AND CREATE SPACE FOR MIRACLES

Carrie Roldan

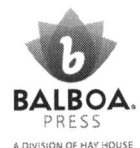

BALBOA.
PRESS
A DIVISION OF HAY HOUSE

Balboa Press books may be ordered through booksellers or by contacting:

Balboa Press
A Division of Hay House
1663 Liberty Drive
Bloomington, IN 47403
www.balboapress.com
1 (877) 407-4847

Because of the dynamic nature of the Internet, any web addresses or links contained in this book may have changed since publication and may no longer be valid. The views expressed in this work are solely those of the author and do not necessarily reflect the views of the publisher, and the publisher hereby disclaims any responsibility for them.

The author of this book does not dispense medical advice or prescribe the use of any technique as a form of treatment for physical, emotional, or medical problems without the advice of a physician, either directly or indirectly. The intent of the author is only to offer information of a general nature to help you in your quest for emotional and spiritual well-being. In the event you use any of the information in this book for yourself, which is your constitutional right, the author and the publisher assume no responsibility for your actions.

Any people depicted in stock imagery provided by Thinkstock are models, and such images are being used for illustrative purposes only. Certain stock imagery © Thinkstock.

Printed in the United States of America.

ISBN: 978-1-4525-9547-4 (sc)
ISBN: 978-1-4525-9548-1 (e)

Library of Congress Control Number: 2014906117

Balboa Press rev. date: 07/03/2014

Forward
By Lisa Engles

Running is my spiritual cardio-therapy. Every time I lace up my shoes to hit the trails in the coastal mountains of the San Francisco Bay Area, I know that I'm not just preparing to exercise. I'm preparing for a conversation with God. I'm ringing the doorbell to the House of the Divine. And I'm stepping into a communion between my body, my mind, and my highest self... literally.

It wasn't always this way. I started running in my freshman year at Huntington Beach High School, in Southern California and immediately became one of the 'stars' on the varsity team. I thrived off of running fast. But I thrived even more off of the attention I got as someone who excelled.

It's not too much of a stretch to say that I was obsessed with running. I started doing double workouts – running on my own before I went to school and again at practice with my team-- in an attempt to get the competitive edge. I even joined a local running team, separate from my high school team, to get trained by one of the area's best coaches.

This obsession followed me into college where I got involved in triathlon, which, to some degree, was a good thing, because after four years of thrashing my body with running, I was constantly riddled with injuries. Triathlon was a band-aid, allowing me to give my body some rest from the effects of being an over-trained runner. The cross-training was good for my body and seemed to bring balance. But before I knew it, I had traded in my obsession with running for an obsession with triathlon. (Can you say A-D-D-I-C-T-I-O-N?)

In total, I was a competitive runner for twenty-two years and a competitive triathlete for seventeen years. By the time I was thirty-three, my body was breaking down to the point of being in constant pain. Having a two-year old daughter, and being in a failing marriage, made matters worse. It's always easier to deal with something like a broken body when you're not also dealing with a broken marriage. Let's just say that I wasn't in a very good place.

I was at a cross roads. The impulse to break free of the pain – physically, mentally and emotionally –- over took me like a tsunami. Something had to fundamentally change within me, and I wasn't going to take 'No' for an answer. That was ten years ago and it all seems like a blur now, but I can remember that there were two things that got me through those times: My relationship with the Divine, and my running practice.

I've always been a spiritual person-- even as a kid, I actually enjoyed... no, I *loved* going to church. And as I got older, I began to explore. I became a spiritual tourist, so to speak. Christianity, New Thought, Buddhism, the teachings of Paramahansa Yoganada. Some form of 'God' always was always present in my life.

During that time, my daily runs turned into my daily prayers. I didn't care how far or how fast I ran. I just knew that I needed to move my body. Running provided a safe-haven. It was familiar, I knew what to expect, and it transported me to a happier place.

Soon, I began to recognize that happy place as a communion with Spirit. The satisfaction of *that* feeling was unparalleled to any feeling I'd ever had in all my years of being a competitive runner and triathlete. All the personal records, all the championship wins... they paled in comparison to the calm inner-peace and deep sense of knowing that I was being held by a Power far beyond my conscious understanding, every time I laced up my running shoes. I had finally found the attention I had been seeking all those years as a young runner, all those years as a high performing triathlete.

I awakened to the Truth that I had heard for so long, but never really heard: Happiness can only come from within. It always sounded so cliché to me. But I got it, and I became passionate about living and teaching that Truth and how to find it through running.

Carrie Roldan's book, *Run Yourself Happy* teaches this fundamental truth in a compassionate, light-hearted, and authentic way. Within moments of meeting Carrie for the first time, I knew that she was a soul (and sole) sister, who shared the same understanding of the power of running as a mindful, meditative practice as opposed to just another activity to cram into your hectic schedule in an effort to stay healthy.

Carrie offers twelve running practices that bridge mind, body, and spirit, creating a truly holistic approach to your daily run. The best part is, you don't have to identify yourself as being a 'runner' to benefit from these practices. By following her simple approach, you'll soon discover that you too can 'run yourself happy' as long as you have a pair of running shoes and an open mind.

Run Yourself Happy is a wonderful resource for anyone who desires to harness the full potential of mind, body and spirit through the activity of running.

Lisa Engles,

Author of Breathe Run Breathe, creator of the Breathe Run Breathe Running Program, Head Running Coach, Silicon Valley Triathlon

For Jim, Quinn, Brady, and Chase.

I love you.

May you each live fully in your soul's calling.

Run Yourself Happy

A FIVE WEEK TRAINING PROGRAM TO RELEASE ANXIETY AND CREATE SPACE FOR MIRACLES

By Carrie Roldan

Preface

The purpose of this book is to help women who run to release anxiety and make space for miracles in their lives. And believe me, no matter where you are right now, if you apply the principles and practical tools offered in this book, your life will absolutely change for the better. I know. It continues to happen for me. Miracles continue to show up in my life in the most wonderfully serendipitous, and totally unexpected, ways.

If I had seen a book like this a year ago, I would have jumped at the chance to read it, because I was in a very different place than I am now. I was a runner who knew I needed to run just to keep myself from going crazy. Running wasn't so much of a happiness practice for me as it was a coping mechanism. I was anxious and stressed most of the time, and I couldn't quite put my finger on *why*. I would not have described myself as *un*-happy, but I was definitely unfulfilled. I was busting at the seams with potential, and could feel that there was something truly great inside of me. I just had no idea what it was.

Money was tight (to say the least), and I struggled to find a sense of worth, while barely making a financial contribution to my family. I was a stay-at-home mom who earned a meager paycheck from a marketing gig for a former employer, and the occasional (okay, truly rare) life coaching client. My marriage was going through a rough patch. This is not to say that we were on the path to divorce; only that I felt unsupported and alone.

I've always been a runner, and over the past decade I've become a total personal and spiritual growth junkie. For the past several years, I've been waking up early to read, meditate, and journal before I start my day. I've practiced the Law of Attraction to great success in certain areas of my life, but seemed absolutely unable to manifest the things that I desperately wanted.

I understood that it was the desperation that stood in my way, but couldn't seem to shake it. I'd catch glimpses of alignment with my highest calling, but they were fleeting and unfocused. I loved the daily practice of intending to connect with my soul, and my mornings were generally glorious! But once the kids woke up, and I busied myself with the tasks of my day, all enlightened action was off. Despite nearly ten years of practice, I still struggled to incorporate what I had learned in my spiritual practice into my "real" life.

Until...

Until one day, I made a conscious decision to run myself happy. I knew that I had the answers somewhere inside of me, and I knew that I had to start applying the principles that I had learned in all of the years of personal development and spiritual growth. So I did what I knew how to do. I ran. And each day on my run, I did an exercise from this book, and an incredibly magnificent shift began to happen inside of me. And then I saw it manifesting in my life. It was so incredibly simple, yet totally life changing.

This book is designed to help you do exactly what I did. I used my daily run as a time to connect with a higher power, and to listen to my intuition; the call of my soul. That's it.

In the pages that follow, I share my story and offer tips, tricks, and techniques that I have used to change my life for the better. I'm now living the life I was too afraid to live just a year ago. I'm playing a much bigger game, because I feel a sense of ease and peace around who I am, what I have to offer, and the impact that I am meant to make on the world. I am truly happy, and I want that for you too.

Contents

PART ONE

Chapter 1
THE SUMMER OF 2013

The summer of 2013 marked a turning point for me. It was the summer that I deliberately ran myself happy. It was the summer that this book whispered itself in my ear, and the exercises within came to me as I ran each day. The summer of 2013 is when I embraced my life's purpose (even though I didn't quite yet understand it), and began the life I had been too afraid to live before. But that isn't to say that it was all sunshine and rainbows. You don't feel the urge to run yourself happy unless you are noticeably *un*-happy!

From the outside looking in, I have always appeared to be "happy." I'm naturally optimistic, and quick to smile or crack a joke. I'm known for being genuine, and am sought after for inspiration and wholehearted support. If you have a dream, I believe in that dream with you, and for you. I hold the vision of your dream even when you have lost sight of it. As a life coach, it is my job to help you to breathe life into that dream. But, by the summer of 2013, I was coming to a "rock bottom" when it came to my own dreams. Funny how that works.

My Dreams

I have always dreamed of being a speaker, author, entrepreneurial muse, and inspiration. I have been a coach for fifteen years; first a cross country and track coach, and later, a life coach. I absolutely *live* to help people to recognize, believe in, and live their potential. I see greatness all around me, and relish helping people to go beyond their expectations and live in the fullness of what they are meant to be doing. My experience as both a NCAA division I athlete and coach has shown me that a strong belief in what's possible, coupled with persistence, can yield "impossible" results. I can literally feel potential in others and have a true gift for nurturing and growing it.

And Yet....

And yet, by the summer of 2013, I was beginning to lose faith in my own dreams. I was generally dissatisfied in several areas of my life. My physical body was beginning to take a shape that I didn't like. I'd always been an athlete, but at thirty-seven and after having three kids, I began to look… well, mom-ish! I recognized my body, but it didn't belong to me. It belonged to the version of my mother that I remember from my childhood.

And my relationship with my husband was less than ideal. I would have called it a "happy" marriage, in the sense that we generally got along, but I felt unsupported in my dreams, and trapped by what I perceived to be his lack of faith in my ability to achieve what, deep down, I knew I was capable of accomplishing.

I loved him, but I desperately needed his approval and support, and was afraid to ask for it, because my inner voice warned me that I wouldn't get it. My fear of his disapproval and/or rejection was driving a wedge between us. Resentment was building on both sides.

To escalate matters, my "career" was stagnant. I put the word *career* in quotations because I barely considered either of my businesses a career. I still answered the question of "what do you do?" with "I'm a stay-at-home-mom, but I also do life coaching, and I have a side business called Dinner This Month." I didn't really consider my businesses my career, but I had completely tied my happiness to the idea that I needed to be a successful entrepreneur. Dinner This Month (a company that my friends and I created and run) was paying its own bills, but not reaching the wider audience that I knew it could serve, and my coaching business was at a standstill. I had had a few successful clients, but had let my web URL lapse, and was doing zero marketing. I knew it was what I was meant to be doing, but also felt that I just didn't have time for it. With three young children, I struggled to find balance. Time for me. Time for my marriage. Time for my businesses. My life was one long to-do list, and it felt empty, meaningless, and lonely.

The Other Thing

And there was this other thing. This part of me that felt like a fraud. I spent so much time and energy believing in other people's dreams, and helping them to take the steps necessary to achieve them, but I was struggling to live my own. I was so busy just keeping up with the laundry, play dates, and day-to-day tasks, that I had lost touch with my purpose, my intuition, and my dreams. My dream was to be a successful author, speaker, coach, and entrepreneur. I dreamed of using my gifts and talents to serve the world on a bigger scale.

I wanted to make a big impact. But I was living a scattered life. Three young children on summer break and an aggressive travel schedule, on a very limited budget, left me feeling depleted and hopeless. I had this instinctive knowing that I was at a turning point. If I didn't do something *now*, I would continue to sink into the half- life that I was already living. If I didn't take action toward my dream life, I was going to settle for who I currently was, and never step into the life I knew I was meant to live. It was time to be brave; to "go big or go home."

The trouble was, I didn't know what action to take. I didn't know what I didn't know. I just knew that the more I continued to live the way I was living, the less authentic I felt. And for someone who counts authenticity in her top five values, this was an unbearable disappointment. And the worst part was that I blamed my husband and my children for my state. Not directly, of course, but I used them and their needs as an excuse not to live fully.

Perhaps my biggest excuse, however, was "not enough money." My limiting beliefs about money have played a massive role in my life until now. I blamed my lack of action on the idea that we couldn't afford, or worse, that Jim (my husband) wouldn't *allow* me to spend on products or services that would help me to further my dreams. I was sitting in a self imposed prison of inaction, excuses, victimhood, and limiting beliefs. Not exactly a winning combination. And, as someone who calls herself a life coach, it was time for me to start walking my talk!

I Committed to Living My Purpose

So, I made a commitment. I committed to myself. I committed to listening to the call of my soul, to trusting that I am guided by a force greater than myself, and to following the guidance that arrived. Honestly, I'm not sure where this commitment came from. I think it came from deep within me. Maybe from lifetimes ago. But it was strong. It was brave. It was a stubborn child who refused to accept less than she deserved. It was a part of me that I barely recognized, but at the same time, I knew. I knew this voice. I knew this girl. I knew that whatever I was about to do *must* be done. I just had no idea what it was that I was about to do. I was terrified.

My great big fear was that I would have to leave my husband in order to find myself and live my purpose. I had projected all of my limiting beliefs onto him, and he personified the oppressive force of all of my fears. Would I need to leave him to live the life I knew I was meant to lead? I decided that I needed to be brave enough to find out.

Deep down, I knew that Jim was not my real problem, but I had to be willing to accept that he might not be along for the ride. I made a commitment to living the life that was inside of me. The life that was aching to be lived. And while I was petrified, I was also empowered. Deciding is a powerful thing.

I had no idea what to do, and only a vague inkling of what my purpose was. I just knew that I couldn't live the hum-drum "good" life that I was already living. And it was, by all standards, a good life. We have a nice home that we can afford. We live in a good neighborhood with awesome neighbors. Our three kids are happy and healthy, and I'm able to stay home with them while they are young. But, I needed great. I needed fulfilling. I needed purposeful, abundant, joyful, and prosperous. I needed more. I couldn't call myself "happy" because I wasn't fulfilled. And I was nowhere near peaceful. I was anxious, afraid, and ambitious.

The Winds of Change

Early in the summer of 2013, my family took our yearly vacation. One of the best things Jim and I have done as a couple was to buy a timeshare on our honeymoon in Cabo San Lucas, Mexico. It forces us to take a very nice vacation each year, which we would otherwise not be able to afford. But, more than that, it allows us to rest and luxuriate for an entire week, focusing on nothing else but what feels right for that particular day. This year's vacation was one of our best. We barely left the resort, and spent a lot of time napping. One morning, though, as I sat alone on the balcony listening to the rhythmic whooshing of the crashing waves, and writing in my journal, I felt the change.

There was a change in the usually dry desert air. It was sticky, tropical, and windy. A storm was approaching and I felt the winds of change. A voice whispered in my ear; not an audible voice from outside my head, but *my* voice, only coming from somewhere else. It whispered what I already knew. These were the winds of change. These winds would deliver a storm, but after the storm, the clouds would clear, and life would be refreshed, brilliant, and spectacular.

In that moment, I surrendered. I asked for guidance and sat in a place of knowing that it would arrive. I decided that I would choose to believe that whatever showed up in my life, or in my heart, was placed there by a benevolent force greater than me, and that my job was to accept it, and to act on it. As Louise Hay says, my job was to "do what was in front of me." But what showed up was not what I expected. It was a storm of emotion. Of fear. Of anger. Of dissatisfaction. I was faced with the fact that I've lived most of my adult life on the verge.

Guidance

What arrived was a desire to run on a daily basis, and to read three books. I'm a Facebook fan of Wayne Dyer, and when I returned from vacation, I saw a post of his recommending a book that he was currently working through. It was called E^2, and without much thought, I followed the Amazon.com link and purchased the Kindle copy.

I had ordered Gabrielle Bernstein's *May Cause Miracles* a few months prior, and had made an attempt to read it in early April. But I just couldn't. It felt overwhelming and exhausting. But when I returned from vacation, I noticed it again, and took this as a sign that it was time to open it and get reading.

The third book that appeared in my life that summer was Brené Brown's *Daring Greatly*. I can't remember exactly when I ordered it, but I have been slowly reading it for several months. This is unusual for me as I tend to devour books, but *Daring Greatly* is different for some reason. I picked it up in the summer of 2013, and continue to read it, on and off, as I write. I can tell you this, though, each time I pick it up, it speaks to where I currently am, and offers wisdom, perspective, and clarity. I have surrendered to the fact that I don't need to push myself through *Daring*

Greatly, and that it will call to me when I am ready or willing to receive what it has to offer.

A fourth book arrived a little later. It actually showed up right after school started in September, but it made a big impact. Fabienne Fredrickson's *Embrace Your Magnificence* spoke right to my heart and empowered me to face my demons and walk my talk in a big way. Working the principles in that book as I continued to work through *May Cause Miracles* helped me to reclaim myself, love my life, find true happiness, and write this book.

A Commitment to Daily Running

So, I was unhappy. I felt depressed about the shape and feel of both my body and my marriage. I felt detached from myself. Running has always been a part of my life, and it is something that generally helps my happiness factor. But I committed to running because I know how to do that. I know how to commit to a daily training regimen. I'd been a competitive runner through high school and college and had coached runners for ten years after. Committing to running was comfortable. It was safe. It was easy for me to do.

A Commitment to Walking My Talk

I'm great at concepts. I get things on an intellectual level really easily. I can articulate theories and principles from sunup to sundown. I *love* to live in the space of what is possible. But action, implementation, actually *doing* the things necessary for change and development? Well, that was a bit scarier. I preferred to hide behind the excuses I have already mentioned... my husband and kids. Oh, and the lack of money.

A Journey of A Thousand Miles Begins With a Single Step

But I took the first step. I read all of the books that arrived and combined their wisdom with what I had learned over the past decade as a personal growth junkie and spiritual seeker. And lo and behold, miracles happened. Little by little, and sometimes all at once, I ran myself happy. It has been a truly miraculous transformation, and one that I am eager to share with you.

Chapter 2
HOW CAN I SERVE?

"How Can I Serve?"

"How can I serve?" This is a spiritual mantra as well as an enlightened entrepreneur's saying that I hear often. And I get it... Give, and you shall receive. Serve your clients well, and you shall be richly rewarded. But I gotta tell ya, I have really struggled with it. I struggle because I *do* want to serve, but I also want to be *paid* for my work and for my time... and I have had a really hard time, in the past, doing both.

So, I began to take this mantra with me out on my runs. "How can I serve?" Honestly, it took a while for me to get this one. Because the answers didn't come as words in my head. They came later, as opportunities in my life. And soon after, I encountered a slightly different variation in my reading of Gabrielle Bernstein's *May Cause Miracles:* "I am here to be truly helpful."

Answering the first question of "How can I serve?" didn't give me the instant client boost that I wanted. Instead, this book began whispering itself in my ear. Truthfully, it took me a long time to put the two together. I have always been a writer, and have wanted to be an author since I can't even remember. There are lots of books inside of me, and I was actually in the middle of writing one, when this little guy interrupted and pressed itself upon my consciousness. But, it answers that fundamental question of "How can I serve?" This book is one of the many answers that I received while doing what I offer in the pages that follow. I am reminded that I am here to be truly helpful, and now understand that my happiness, and my success are tied to one another, but they are not the same thing.

So, before you read on, ask yourself this: "How can I serve?" Place it in your consciousness as you head out on today's (or tomorrow's) run. And look for opportunities to be of service. Pick up litter that you see. Help a person who asks for directions. Offer words of encouragement to other runners. But also, be still (well, internally still) and listen. Listen to your intuition. Is it nudging you to call a friend? Write a thank you letter? Order a product?

And be open. Be open throughout your day. Be open to rearranging your schedule based on what appears in your experience on your run. Remember, you are here to be truly helpful. Let this guide you as you run, as you read on, and as you live your life.

Chapter 3
WHY RUNNING?

It should be clear from a book entitled *Run Yourself Happy* that some running is going to be involved. But *why* running? Why use the one thing that more sports offer as punishment than anything else, as a happiness tool? Well, if you are already a runner, you know the answer to this question. Running is more than just running. And, while runners don't always have a smile on their face *during* our runs, we are a generally happy, up-beat group. If you have any doubts, go and check out the start line of a marathon on any given Saturday or Sunday at the butt-crack of dawn. Or better yet, head to the finish line!

And running seems to create community, which is a very basic human need. It is totally normal to find groups of runners gathered at parks, trailheads, running stores, and the like. We meet with each other to share the experience of running in community. And there are scores of online running communities as well. Runners seek each other out and naturally form communities based the basic human need for community, and the shared experience of running.

It's Science

The physical act of running is really pretty cool. While it seems counterintuitive that running for miles on end would induce the brain and body's pleasure response, it turns out to be true. Most people have heard about the endorphin release triggered by running. Endorphins are proteins produced by the endocrine system that are often described as "natural pain killers." They cause a natural sense of well being. But new research also connects running to serotonin and dopamine release. These are neurotransmitters associated with mood regulation and reward-motivated behavior. So, while I don't pretend to understand all of the ins and outs of the science, it is important to note that the act of running produces chemical responses in the body that help you feel good.

Full Disclosure: I know that there is a ton of empirical data on the correlation between running and happiness. And there is even an emergent branch of psychotherapy called "running therapy." But, since experience speaks much louder than a Google search, I think it is best to share what I know from experience.

Running is More Than Running

Running is more than just running. It's more than one foot in front of the other, breathe in, breathe out. Something *happens* on a run. Something beyond endorphins and neurotransmitters. Something spiritual. For me, running has been a lot of things over the course of my life, but one thing is for certain, it has always been more than just running.

The act of running breathes into my soul. It speaks to my dreams, my desires, and my heart. Running gives birth to my creativity, and puts my mind right. I release anger, frustration, doubt, and worry, and make way for miracles. No matter how big the problem, I always feel better about it after a run. Running is meditation in motion, and it has become my daily happiness practice.

What Running Will Do For You

Chances are, if you are reading this book, you already have an inkling that running can help you to get your life on track. But running itself is not necessarily enough. You must choose to turn your daily run into your daily happiness practice. Yes, I said "daily"… twice. But don't freak out if you aren't a daily runner yet. You will be soon. You will look forward to it. You'll start to need it. Running with the practices laid out in this book will absolutely create the space in your life for miracles to occur.

Yes, I said "miracles." Don't freak out about that either. I'm not talking the parting of the Red Sea, but trust me on this one. They will occur. They will likely start out quite small. Hardly noticeable, even. But as you notice, they will grow incrementally. Then they will snowball, and before you know it, you'll be living a full blown miracle.

So what does it mean to be living a full blown miracle? It's friggin' awesome! For me, it is living my life's purpose, understanding my unique gifts, and sharing them with the world. It feels *incredible*, and I absolutely want this same feeling for you.

How to Get Your Full Blown Miracle

I've heard faith defined as "believing in that which you cannot see." And while I know that a miracle is defined by *A Course In Miracles* as "a shift in perception," I think a full blown miracle occurs when you let go of the "how" attached to your dreams or goals, you choose to have *faith* in them. When this happens, miracles occur naturally. So, in case you missed the three steps to full blown miracle creation, here they are:

1. *Release the "how" attached to your dream, goal, or desire.* In other words, let go of the way that you think it would have to happen. Or more likely, why you think it is nearly impossible.

2. *Choose to have faith.* Faith doesn't mean religion. It means *belief.* It means deciding to believe in that thing that you have absolutely no idea how to make happen. This is no small choice. It means bypassing all logic, and believing anyway. Faith is easier if you *feel* your way there.

3. *Miracles start to occur.* They may not look like the full blown miracle that you have envisioned, but as you notice the small miracles in your life, they will build momentum.

There is something truly magical that happens on a run; a momentum that literally creates the space for this process to occur. The conscious mind seems to tire with the body, and an open, creative, and receptive spiritual space becomes accessible. You will use the activities in this book to capitalize on that spiritual space.

My Running Journey

I've been a runner since I was fourteen years old. I fell into running, actually. I had been a competitive gymnast for several years, but I was over 5'5" tall, and had stopped improving. At age fourteen, I let go of my dream of becoming the next Mary-Lou Retton, and began my search for the next athletic endeavor to occupy my time. I was either going to join the cross country team, or become a competitive weight lifter. For anyone who knows me, or has seen my physique, the weight lifter thing is beyond hilarious. But, I was totally serious at the time. Since my high school had a cross country team, and because they didn't want me to become all self-obsessed and muscle bound, my parents encouraged me to join cross country. Good call, Bob and Gayle. I'm glad I listened.

This decision impacted my life in ways that are still manifesting. I've been a runner ever since. Running led me to my husband, whom I met on the cross country team at UC Irvine, and to a career as a cross country and track coach, first at the high school level, and later as a volunteer assistant at the University of California, Irvine. But running has been different things at different times in my life.

The Roles of Running

At fourteen, running was belonging. Being a part of a team felt good, and realizing that I had some talent felt great too. I enjoyed working hard, but it was being part of the team that really mattered at the time. Running was community. It was a place to be accepted, and to belong. Running was very social at fourteen.

Later, running was goal setting and achievement. It is easy to measure your improvement and success at running, because the watch doesn't lie. Running was a place where I could experiment with life. I learned that hard work does pay off, but that too much leads to exhaustion and injury. I learned to have faith in the plan, and believe that great things were possible, even if I had no control over what others did.

Running has been a means to an end for me as well. It helped me to get into college, and has helped me to maintain a healthy weight ever since.

Running has always been a place to think. I've never had much luck with "sleeping on it", but "running on" a problem, or big decision, has always brought me clarity and focus.

But the biggest thing that running has become in my life is a happiness practice. I didn't know it at first. I thought I was running to be healthy, to stay fit, to achieve my goals, or simply because I felt I "should." But after I stopped coaching cross country and track (when my third child was born), I had to find a new reason to run. It was no longer my job to be at practice. Would I choose to run even though I wasn't training for anything? Or training anyone else for anything? Would I still choose to run even though I rarely had anyone else to run with?

At first, I didn't run regularly. It was hard to find the time. My husband insisted that I didn't run alone in the dark, so that meant trying to squeeze in a run sometime after dropping the older kids off at school and before the baby needed to eat. Running was inconvenient, and therefore my runs became inconsistent. Plus, running when you're out of shape is an exercise in frustration. Carrying twenty extra pounds and pushing the baby jogger only added insult to injury. I was slow, heavy, and uncomfortable. So, I chose more convenient mommy-workouts. Yoga, P90X, and Jillian Michaels DVDs became my new workout methodology.

That's when I knew. I knew I needed running to be happy. I was getting fit in my living room, but something was missing. Something primal. Something basic. Something that I only experience while running outdoors. And when I took my spiritual practice on the run, miracles really did happen. And they're still happening!

Running is Good for You

Much of the content of this book will be about the power of personal belief. So, before I go on about the benefits of running, I'd like you to consider what you believe about it. Do you think running is good for you? Do you believe it is an activity that you can continue to do as you age? Or do you believe that running actually ages you? That it wears down your joints and causes foot, knee, and hip ailments?

The truth is, that no matter what your experience until this point may have been to the contrary, we are born to run. It's basic to being human. And while there are plenty who believe that a lifetime of running will cause wear and tear issues in the body, I believe that's just not the case. The wear and tear issues from running don't come from running itself, but from running with improper alignment and muscular imbalances caused from spending much of our days sitting, or doing repetitive movements in our jobs. These can be prevented through proper alignment practices (which I'll help you with in a forthcoming chapter) and nutrition. Science now tells us that load bearing exercise is good for our bones and joint health, and guess what? Running is load bearing.

So, what if you changed the way you thought about running? What if, with every step you took, you chose to believe that you were improving joint health and bone strength? What if, instead of worrying about stress fractures and knee pain, you chose to believe that your daily run would help you to stay vital into old age, and avoid arthritis and osteoporosis? What if you adopted an alignment practice before running that not only helped you feel better, stronger, and more efficient during your run, but also helped you to feel more centered, grounded, and in touch with your true self all day long?

So, Why Running?

Running is an incredible tool for personal and spiritual growth because it connects body and mind. If forces you to hang out with yourself, to push through discomfort, and to surrender to where you are right now. Running is a metaphor for life. And, like happiness, it is a deliberate daily practice. Going on a run is a choice you make on a daily basis. Yes, having a partner or a team to run with helps. So does having a coach, or a training program; but ultimately, the choice to run is yours, and owning this choice makes all of the difference. Your happiness is no different. It helps to have accountability buddies, a coach, and a plan, but ultimately, the choice is yours. Choose happiness.

Chapter 4

DECIDE TO BE HAPPY

Before you read on, I need for you to do something for me. I need for you to decide to be happy. Decide that happiness is possible for you; that the life you're longing for *is* possible, even if you can't possibly see how. This is so important because, unless you do this one thing, the rest of this book is just feel-good advice. And while I'm aware that feel-good advice sells books, I'm looking to do a lot more than just sell books. I want this book to make an impact in your life. I want these practices to be a catalyst for real and lasting change.

My intention in writing this book is to share what I have learned and to help you, but it's bigger than that too. I want to create a movement of empowered women who run! I can see you all now, gathering at running shops, parking lots, and trailheads. I see your smiling faces, and can literally feel your empowered and encouraging energy. And how do you create a movement, you ask? One transformation at a time, my friend. One transformation at a time.

We all know the saying, "You can lead a horse to water, but you can't make him drink." The practices in this book *will* make a difference in your life, whether or not you decide to "drink," but for real transformation to occur, you've gotta be willing. I'm going to ask you do so some pretty far-out stuff, but if you are willing, and if you are committed to your own full-blown miracle life, then you can have it! Remember, you don't have to understand how. Heck, I barely understand how. But that doesn't matter. What matters is that this process is truly transformational, and the *first step* in your transformation is the decision to transform.

Decide to be Happy

You can *want* to be happy until the cows come home, but if you don't believe that you're worthy and deserving of happiness, it will always be elusive. If you don't make a *decision* to be happy, you won't be. Now, don't worry, you don't have to feel worthy and deserving just yet. This book will absolutely help with that, but you must decide that you are worth working on, and that happiness is attainable, even for you.

Take my word for it. You deserve to be happy. You were created to live this life in all of its richness and fullness. You were designed to live your highest calling, to share your unique gifts, and to enjoy the process. Happiness is your birthright. So commit to it now.

Decide to be happy.

Now That That's Out of the Way...

Once you've made the decision, commit to doing everything that this book asks of you. You are worth the effort. The mere fact that you are holding this book in your hands (or reading it on a screen) means that this process is part of the unfolding of your life's purpose. There are no accidents. Trust that this has come to you for a reason. Trust that taking action now will lead you in the direction that you need to go.

Go ahead and breathe that in for a moment. It's powerful stuff!

And when you're ready, move on.

Now we've got to deconstruct your idea of what happiness is.

Chapter 5
I'LL BE HAPPY WHEN…

Here's something you might not have considered, but it's the truth, so I feel obliged to tell you: What you think will make you happy, won't.

I really hate to tell you this, but that thing you're chasing, the thing that you just know will make all of the difference for you... well, it won't. Bummer, right? If you think that you'll be happy when you win the lottery, land the dream job, reach your ideal weight, get married or find your dream relationship, or just get your kids to behave, or whatever... you won't. No matter what it is that you think will bring you happiness, I can promise you this, it absolutely will not. There is nothing outside of you that can ever bring you happiness. At least not *real* happiness.

Then why the heck am I writing this book?!?!? Because, I know a secret. I know that happiness is a choice, and that it is an inside job. I know that while there isn't a "thing" that will bring you

25

happiness, there are daily practices that can help you to cultivate it. I know that running is a big part of my personal happiness, and I believe that my experience is universal. I also know that once you cultivate happiness, miraculous shifts occur in all areas of your life.

So, the idea that you'll be happy when you meet Mr. Right is backward. You'll meet Mr. Right once you get happy. Those stubborn ten pounds? They won't stay off until you apply the principles in this book and learn to be happy, no matter what.

I can hear the protests now. "Carrie, I get that. I see that for most areas of my life, but in this one area (money, relationship, body image, career, etc...), I just can't be happy without _____."

"But I know that if I can just find the right relationship, I really *will* be happy."

or

"But I *will* be happy once I am successful and wealthy."

Again, I would like to gently offer that, while I can completely identify with these statements (in fact, at one time in my life or another, I too have believed that once I "got" these things, I would be happy), I can promise that the opposite is true. You will not be able to accept, receive, and enjoy whatever it is you that believe you want *until* you are happy. You will literally be blocking it from your experience.

Do you know how I know that these things won't make you happy? Because you believe that your happiness is contingent upon them. Because you feel incomplete without these things. Or whatever is on your happiness list.

So let's start with your happiness list. What is it that you perceive you need?

Respect?

Money?

Marriage?

Children?

A bigger house?

A better neighborhood?

Success?

What do you feel incomplete without?

Take a few minutes before you read on, and write down the missing pieces to your happiness puzzle. Use a journal, scrap paper, the notes section of your phone, whatever, but write it down. It is very important that you name the things that you believe will fill the emptiness.

Seriously. Do it now. What do you need in order to feel happy? Content? Satisfied with your life? What is missing now? Finish this sentence:

"I know that I would be happy with my life if I could just _____."

I know it seems really real to you. I know that you absolutely believe that this external thing (or several) will make you happy.

It feels so incredibly real and necessary to your life's satisfaction, but I promise you, it's an illusion. Allow me to explain:

Changing the Illusion

I once believed that I would be happy once I found Mr. Right. Then Jim and I started seriously dating, and I was happy for a while. But before long, the nagging, unfulfilled, empty longing crept back in. Then, I thought I would be happy when we got engaged. And I was for a while. Then, I thought I could finally feel satisfied when we got married... bought a house... had children.... and I was, for a while. But soon I wanted a bigger house, in a better neighborhood, with a pool. I seemed to have a consistent need to fill an ever-growing hole inside me. Can you relate?

Until I became a stay-at-home-mom, I believed that being able to stay home with my kids would be the ultimate "happy" lifestyle. But it wasn't. Suddenly, I believed that a high paying career and more time away from my kids would make me happy. If I just had a nanny... If only I could build a successful business... if only, if only.... Can you see the pattern? I kept getting the things that I thought would make me happy, but happiness was still elusive. And I'm betting that you can tell a very similar story.

I had the life I thought I wanted, and I still felt unfulfilled.

Here's the problem: the story we tell ourselves about happiness... It's a lie!

So let me explain what I mean by "happy." Many pretty amazing people, spiritual gurus, and personal growth experts make a distinction between happiness and joy. *Happiness*, they say, is fleeting; a temporary emotional state brought about by external circumstances. While *joy* is an internal condition; a state of being. And it is this internal state of being that we all seek when we look for "happy."

Why, then, have I titled this book "Run Yourself Happy"? Well, because in our culture, we chase happiness in search of joy, contentment, satisfaction, and peace. So, what I propose is that, for the purposes of this book, we consider "happy" as the ideal of peaceful, purposeful, contented, satisfied, and any other adjective that suits you. We're not looking for the fleeting moment of happiness brought about by external circumstances. We're going to do the work to cultivate a happy life; one filled with the pervading internal states of joy, gratitude, and peace.

If you do the practices in this book, you will find that you are happier. And because you are happier, you will get the things you thought would make you happy in the first place. Capicé? It may feel counterintuitive, but it's true. Happiness comes from within. It comes from choosing to love yourself and know that you are worthy, deserving, and *enough*.

PART TWO

Chapter 6
HOW TO USE THIS BOOK

Congratulations on making the decision to Run Yourself Happy! Whether you are new to running, and looking for a vehicle to get in shape and boost your endorphins, or you are already a runner looking for more happiness in your life, you've come to the right place. This five week plan will guide you through the steps of self discovery, awareness, and action necessary to live your "full blown miracle" life.

Before We Get Started:

The program that I am about to take you through is both subtle and powerful. It is designed to help you get out of your own way, and open you up to the life that you desire and deserve. And, while I know that the simple act of running can make a huge difference in your overall happiness quotient, running through the steps that I will guide you through will be absolutely life altering. At the end of five weeks, you will be aligned with the life that you are meant to be living.

A Few Commitments

For you to get the most out of this book, you will need to commit to the following:

1. Trust the Process

While the work you will be doing is mostly internal, and generally subtle, gentle, and empowering, it is also both powerful and intense. You will be clearing away some old, negative energy and thought patterns, and making space for greatness. I ask that you honor yourself and whatever comes up, and that you trust the process enough to continue your daily Run Yourself Happy practices.

2. Keep an Open Mind

This goes hand in hand with trusting the process. I am going to be asking you to do some things that may look or feel silly, for reasons that may seem absolutely ridiculous given your current mindset. My request is that you keep your heart and mind open enough to try them. I promise that you have nothing to lose.

3. Run 4X per Week or More

I've designed the content of this book with the "daily run" in mind. While I am a huge proponent of rest and recovery, I also believe that it is essential that you commit to running more days than you don't. In a seven day week, that means at least four days. Ideally, you will run six days and rest on the seventh. But, if you are not in shape to actually run that many days in a row, it is important to get out the door and jog, or power-walk, on the days that running feels impossible. You'll also notice that each chapter has only three daily practices. This is intentional, as they are "practices" and therefore ought to be *practiced* more than once. Simply repeat the Run Yourself Happy practices that feel right, or that you find exceptionally helpful.

4. Run Outside

There's no denying the link between cardiovascular activity and increased feelings of well being. I'm not talking "runner's high" here. Cardio (running or not) increases serotonin levels, which leads to warm fuzzies. But, running is somehow different. It's magical. It has healing powers.

Now, let me be clear about one thing: when, I talk about running, I always mean "running outdoors." Treadmill running falls into the "cardio" category. I'm blessed in that I live in Southern California, and can run outdoors all year long, but before you start whining about how cold it can get where you live, let me just share that I've spoken to high school teams from Alaska, North Dakota, and upstate New York who all run outside in some pretty gnarly conditions. The Alaskan team's coach put drywall screws through the bottom of their training shoes so they could get traction on the frozen ground. "training spikes," in essence.

When I was shivering in the dreary forty degree weather in Portland, Oregon, the team from North Dakota shared with me that they train outside unless the temperature dips below -20°. That's twenty degrees below zero, people! And these are ninety-five pound high school girls! The point is, running outside can happen for much of the year, no matter where you live. Running on a treadmill just isn't the same. Please make every attempt to get outside as often as possible.

Now, sure, I'm using examples of competitive athletes, but anyone who has ever been a runner knows the difference. Fresh air matters. Change of scenery matters. And I believe that these things are absolutely part of the happiness factor.

Plenty of studies exist on the psychological benefits of experiencing nature. And, while I know that there are treadmills that can be programmed to show you scenes of nature on a video screen, it simply doesn't compare to actually being outside. You don't have to be outside on picturesque mountain trail, or running along beautiful beaches. Pounding the pavement in suburbia counts as nature too! There are benefits to breathing fresh air, feeling the cold (or heat), noticing the sky, the birds, the trees, the cars... all of it.

I don't want to belabor the point, but let's just come to an understanding that for the purposes of this book, "running" means *running outside*. Anything else falls into the "cardio" category.

5. Journal

Each Run Yourself Happy practice has some post-run journal questions at the end. It's up to you whether you decide to spend time journaling immediately post-run, or sometime later in the day. I like to journal immediately after a run because it is when

I feel the most open, inspired, and creative. However, bedtime is also a great time to journal and reflect on the growth and lessons of the day.

The journal questions are meant to help you get started, and once you start, the ideas will flow. Commit to journaling at least fifteen minutes per day. This practice alone could radically affect your happiness quotient. The simple act of getting thoughts out of your head, and onto paper, can be powerful and transformative. And, because you will be keeping a record, you'll be able to track your progress. A journal is a tangible way to see just how far you've come, so please don't skip this step.

Here's how it Works:

The chapters are divided into weeks, and each week has a theme that will contribute to your overall happiness, and Run Yourself Happy exercises that compliment the theme. However, there are two practices that ought to be incorporated at least once per week, every week. These are "Alignment," and "Run with a Friend." I'll explain these first, before the Week 1 chapter.

Please read the chapter introductions at your leisure, but do your best to read (or at least review) the Run Yourself Happy practices immediately prior to heading out the door for your run. As the weeks progress, you may want to repeat, or layer, the practices. This is encouraged. At first, what I suggest will take deliberate focus on your part, but at the end of the five weeks, you may notice that they are second nature. You'll enjoy a new way of being, and a totally new appreciation for your daily runs.

Let's Do This!

I know that if you can stick with it, and run at least four days a week, while doing the practices I lay out for you, for the next five weeks, you'll experience a miraculous happiness shift. So, thanks for playing along. It's going to be life changing. Woohoo!!! Let's get started.

Chapter 7
ALIGNMENT

Alignment is more than just posture, and takes more than a few chiropractic adjustments. Alignment is both physical and spiritual. To truly be happy, one must align their thoughts, actions, and behaviors with their values. I have a saying that I used to tell the girls that I coached: "behave like the person you hope to become." I think I may have stolen this from John Maxwell, but it has become a driving force in my life. I often ask myself, what would Ideal Me do?

Ideal Me

Ideal Me is gentle. She forgives. She has compassion. She takes risks because she isn't afraid to fail. Ideal Me fully inhabits herself, and loves herself and others unconditionally. She is truly aligned with her life's purpose and profits from it greatly. She acts from a belief in who she is, and what she stands for.

And guess, what? Ideal Me exists! And I chose to become her (or not), more and more each day, with every choice I make.

I have spent the past several years working at getting into alignment. This has meant working at getting my thoughts, behaviors, and decisions in alignment with what my gut tells me, with my intuition, and with the call of my soul. I've read more self-help than I previously knew existed, and have worked with coaches and intuitives to help shepherd me along my path.

I've learned a lot over the course of my journey, but perhaps the most profound lesson is this: *true happiness cannot exist outside of alignment.* In other words, you cannot enjoy your life if you are not living it in alignment with your values, and your purpose. You may attain the life you thought, or were taught, that you wanted, but without alignment, it will feel empty and unfulfilling.

Life Is Symbolic

The thing about life, is that it is just so amazingly symbolic. It's truly awesome, beautiful, and perfect that getting into proper physical alignment can actually help you to align energetically with your spirit. The mind/body connection is widely accepted in the scientific and medical communities. We understand that stress decreases our immune response, and can lead to all sorts of undesirable medical conditions. We also understand that simple breathing, and mental exercises, can help to reduce stress. Most people also recognize that we hold stress in various parts of our bodies. You can probably attest to having had a stress knot in your neck or shoulders, or feeling tightness in your jaws during times of extreme stress.

Oftentimes, holding stress in our bodies can keep us out of alignment with our Ideal Selves, our spirits, and our souls. When we choose to hold on to anger, resentment, blame, and the like, we choose to cut ourselves off from our true nature. Feeding our anger is like taking poison and expecting the other person to die. Our anger, resentment, judgment, etc, doesn't harm the other person, but it does keep us from alignment with our Ideal Self. I'm assuming, here, that judgment and anger aren't part of your core values. I'm making the leap that these are not things that you would say your Ideal Self stands for. If they are, I'm thinking that this book isn't for you.

When we hold these bad-feeling thoughts and feelings in our bodies for an extended period of time, we don't just fall out of alignment with our Ideal Selves, we also fall out of physical alignment. Our posture suffers. And vice versa. Physical misalignment leads to feeling disconnected from your Ideal Self.

Ideal Me is physically fit, stands tall, and radiates confidence and love. I'm guessing that Ideal You is similar. No one pictures their ideal self as fat, slouchy, and sheepish! But habitually holding poor posture blocks your natural energy flow, and will actually cause you to feel this way.

When we have jobs that cause us to sit for extended periods of time, or have to perform repetitive motions, we often fall out of physical alignment, which can lead to pain. Pain is such a beautiful message from the body. Pain is your body's way of saying, "something's off here. Please stop what you are doing, and adjust." Keyword: adjust.

Mind-Body Alignment

What I have found to be true, is that when I dedicate a portion of my day to getting into proper skeletal alignment, I feel the domino effect. Getting physically aligned leads me to feel more centered, grounded, peaceful, and alive; which, I believe, is energetic alignment with my soul. I feel more peaceful, purposeful, creative, and enthusiastic about my life. This energetic alignment opens the door to my intuition, which helps me to feel guided, spiritually aligned, and connected to all that is. It's amazing what a few minutes of postural alignment work can do to re-connect regular-old-me with Ideal Me. And when I'm connected to Ideal Me, I'm happier because I'm living in alignment with who I *truly* am.

A More Practical Approach for Runners

For those of you who just aren't buying the mind/body thing, there are some really practical reasons to integrate a skeletal alignment practice into your daily Run Yourself Happy practice. The first is injury prevention. By spending a few minutes each day focused on postural alignment, you will be taking massive steps toward injury prevention. Most running injuries can be traced back to muscular imbalances, which are generally rooted in, or caused by, postural imbalances. By spending a few minutes with a daily alignment practice, you'll stretch and straighten the body before you strengthen it.

The second reason that runners need an alignment practice is increased running economy. Running with proper alignment will lead to a more efficient stride, which makes you able to cover more ground with less effort.... which makes you faster!

What is an Alignment Practice?

An alignment practice looks a lot like yoga, or physical therapy exercises; and truthfully, it is both. My friend Laura Jane calls herself a Yoga Therapist, and I believe that she offers the best version of what it is I mean when I say "Alignment Practice." After examining my skeletal imbalances, and listening to my complaints of chronic injuries, Laura Jane devised a "menu" of exercises for me to do, daily, in order to correct them.

Much of this comes from her training as both an Egoscue therapist as well as a yoga instructor. However, what makes the alignment practice so powerful is the intention and breath practices that Laura Jane invites into it. So, while you are working your way through the poses and exercises, you are consciously breathing away resistance, resentments, and impurities. It's powerful work, for both injury prevention, and over-all happiness. I highly recommend that you try incorporating Laura Jane's work into your daily life. At the very least, do it on your days off of running.

I am so passionate about the benefits if Laura Jane's particular brand of yoga therapy, that I have dedicated a whole week of my Run Yourself Happy System online coaching program to it. For more information, visit http://runyourselfhappysystem.com. Laura Jane's website is http://www.ilaurajane.com. She offers a variety of services, including 1:1 consultations and personalized alignment menus designed specifically for you, and your unique imbalances. She has been a godsend in my life, and I am grateful to have found her particular brand of yoga therapy that keeps me feeling aligned, on track, and injury free.

What about Chiropractic Care?

There is absolutely nothing wrong with going to see a chiropractor, but the daily practices that Laura Jane offers may just eliminate the need to go frequently.

What if I Already do Yoga?

Great! Yoga is awesome. And there are about a gazillion different types of yoga practice. Yoga itself is simply a union with all that is, and the postures that we take ourselves through are meant to help the body, mind, and spirit, feel that connection. However, yoga has become a popular workout practice, and if you do it while out of postural alignment, it may actually reinforce imbalances in the same way that running does. It's a good idea to do a little postural therapy before you do your yoga flow class.

Give it a try

Try integrating postural alignment or yoga therapy into your daily life. I suggest using one of Laura Jane's videos, or a personalized practice daily, upon rising, or just before your run. The whole point is to "straighten before you strengthen," and I promise that it will make a world of difference in your life. To learn more about Laura Jane, and her brand of yoga therapy, please visit http://www.ilaurajane.com .

Chapter 8
RUN WITH A FRIEND

This is an easy, yet oh-so-important Run Yourself Happy task. As human beings, we are hard-wired for connection, and we are meant to do life in community. But our world has become one of screens and cubicles, making it easy to avoid actual human interaction. That's why it is so important to deliberately create space for it. Not small talk, but real connection. And what better way to fit it into your busy schedule than on a run?!?

One of the best things about running with a friend, is that it gets "real," quickly. There is something about working out side by side, climbing the same hills, and sweating together that makes space for intimacy and genuine connection. My favorite way to connect with my girlfriends is not to get lunch together, or chat over a cup of coffee; I like to meet up for a run. Meeting at the crack of dawn, with messy hair, mismatched clothes, and the intention to connect, removes all pretenses, and eliminates the need for small talk. We get running, and get to talking about what is important in our lives. Our areas of struggle, our proud moments, the things we are afraid of, whatever is pressing on our hearts at the time, is what comes out on the run. Running with a friend is therapy. It breeds connection, and it's great for the soul.

I laugh and cry while running with friends, and it is always such a cathartic release. Running together creates a sacred space and an intangibly supportive layer to our friendship. It is as if the run symbolizes our resolve to keep going, no matter what is happening in our lives, and to stay side by side. It's a powerful metaphor, and an important message to the Universe.

Choose Wisely

At this point, it is crucial to note, that when I suggest that you run with a friend, it is important that the friend you choose to run with understands that it isn't a race. When you run with a buddy, you are teammates. It's not a competition. You may have to try on several running buddies before you find the right one (or few).

Eventually, your running buddy will become a trusted friend. She will empathize, rather than judge, and offer you love and support, as you run through life together. But take baby steps. I love the way Brené Brown talks about sharing ourselves. She says that we ought only to share our moments of shame and be deeply vulnerable with those who "have earned the right to hear our story." In other words, don't bare your dirty laundry and spill all of your secrets to someone who hasn't yet shown you that she is a loving guardian of your truth. She will reveal her true nature over time, but give it time.

Running is Not a Time for Gossip

Truth be told, there is never a time for gossip in your happy, whole-hearted, full blown miracle life. If you wouldn't say it if the person was standing in the room, it's better left unsaid. Sure, you can talk about your experiences, but gossip is talking about someone else, and usually in a judgmental way. Besides, hopefully this book will have helped you turn your run into a spiritual practice, and gossip has no place in the sacred realm of spiritual growth. You run with a friend to connect, and you cannot truly connect while talking about others. It may feel that way, but it's not real connection. It's a cheap high, a quick fix to generate false intimacy, and it'll leave you feeling depleted. So don't do it.

My Running Buddies

I have three friends that I run with regularly: Jamie, Amy, and Holiday. Jamie is a long-distance BFF because she lives several states away. We see each other a few times a year, and always make time for at least one run together. It never ceases to amaze me that, no matter how much "catching up" we do over the phone, dinner, or vacationing together, the real connecting always happens on our runs. That's where our souls meet and re-connect. The earlier the run happens in our visits, the better time we have, and the more we appreciate our time together.

Holiday is a dear friend from college, and my regular weekend running buddy. She and I know the very best, and very worst, about each other, and each time we run, we choose to let it all hang out. We share our struggles, our fears, and all of the icky sides of ourselves. And we love each other through all of it.

There is something so valuable about running with Holiday, because the act of running brings out the real-ness in each of us. It's hard to feign having it all together as we stumble, slobber, and snot-rocket. The run breaks down all pretenses, and exposes the truth. So we run in truth; we run through physical pain and emotional brokenness. But at the end of the run, we're both still there. Breathing in and out. Side by side. There is something so powerfully supportive, and genuinely comforting about that.

Amy is a former athlete of mine, that I now life coach. I find that our most powerful sessions include a run. Put simply, running is where breakthroughs occur. Holiday has often told me that in order to get clarity on anything, she needs to get her body as tired as her mind. I agree. Physical exhaustion makes room for mental clarity. I see it happen with Amy time and again.

Running lowers her defenses and creates space for miracles... tiny shifts in perception that can change her whole world. And, I find that I am on my best game, as her coach, when I run. Running opens me up too. I feel in my element while running with her, and am able to support her differently. I'm braver in my approach. My defenses and filters dissolve, and I'm able to more deeply connect with my own intuition, which guides the coaching in a truly incredible way. Running together is a powerful practice for both of us.

Why You Gotta

Hopefully all of this talk about intimacy and vulnerability hasn't scared you off! Depending on where you are in your journey, these can sound highly undesirable. But know that they are absolutely necessary for your happiness, as contradictory as that may sound. Brené Brown said, "You cannot get to courage without walking through vulnerability." While I wholeheartedly agree, I also understand that you might not be looking to be courageous. You are, however, human; and humans have a biological need for connectivity. Connection doesn't happen through small talk. It doesn't happen with commiserating either. Connection happens when two souls genuinely show up for each other. And that, my friends, will happen on a run.

At Least Once a Week

So grab a friend. Make a running date, and get your intimacy on. I mean genuine, vulnerable, human interaction. Remember, if the idea of being vulnerable terrifies you, don't stress too much. It will happen little by little. It's not as if going on a run will suddenly crack your protective armor and break you open all at once. But I'll tell you this: if it did, you would feel better. Raw, open, and relieved.

So just do it. Do it because you know it's important, and don't put pressure on yourself to over-share. Just set two very clear intentions:

1. To genuinely show up for your friend. Be the real you. Show real empathy. Experience genuine compassion.

2. To allow yourself to be seen and supported. Receive her friendship and love.

That's it. Just be present and be real, and allow the miracle of human connection to work its magic on your run.

PART THREE

Chapter 9
WEEK 1

Release Stress from the Body

Sometimes it's the simplest things that can initialize the most radical change. This week we are going to release bodily stress, and cultivate calm, ease, and joy. Let's face it, happiness and anxiety cannot coexist. So, as we move into week one of this program, we are going to implement some truly simple strategies to create more calm in your life.

If you suffer from anxiety, you feel it in your body. It sits in your gut like a nervous weight. It churns. This week's activities are both mental and physical, but they are subtle, and easy to implement, and will help to lift the churning, anxious weight in your gut. Everything that you learn this week can, and should, be continued as the weeks progress.

Lasting change doesn't happen by pushing. It happens through a process of opening up and allowing. That is what week one is all about. You will be practicing diaphragmatic breath, relaxing your body, and creating a sense of ease.

This chapter contains three critical Run Yourself Happy practices that are an important foundation for the transformative work that you will be doing over the next five weeks. They are simple, easy to implement, and will become second nature as the weeks progress. As you work through the coming weeks, you will take these practices with you.

This week you'll learn the Mudra Run, The Chest Alive exercise, and my personal favorite, the Horse-Duck-Dog exercise. Despite the fact that you may be running with new physical and mental practices, I believe that you will find this week's Run Yourself Happy practices both enjoyable, and rewarding. And, I assure you, even these very simple practices will radically up your happiness quotient.

As with every week in the program, you will have three new practices introduced. Since it is my expectation that you run at least four times per week, the forth practice could be your run with a friend, or you could choose to do one of these practices more than once. Or, you may simply choose to run with no happiness agenda on the fourth, fifth, or sixth runs of the week.

Just be sure that you continue to do some form of alignment practice throughout. As we have discussed, this will help to keep you in physical alignment, which is important for injury prevention, but there is a spiritual component as well. Trust me on this. You will begin to notice as the weeks progress.

Alright! I'm excited for you... Enjoy!

MUDRA RUN

Today we'll be using a simple mudra to promote deep, full breathing, which, in turn, will create a sense of ease and calm. You cannot expect to feel happy and stressed at the same time, so today's mudra run is designed to help alleviate stress and make way for happiness.

What is a Mudra, Anyway?

I Googled it, and here's what Wikepedia has to say:

> mu·dra
>
> **1**. A symbolic hand gesture used in Hindu and Buddhist ceremonies and statuary, and in Indian dance.

But What Does This Have to do With Running?

Today you are going to practice the mudra for connectivity on your run. The mudra for connectivity is simple. Gently touch the index finger and thumb, like you are making the "OK" symbol. The rest of your fingers should remain relaxed and slightly open. This is a very familiar pose to most yogis, and is often encouraged for meditation.

This mudra is especially important for people who run, because it serves two specific functions. The first is to keep the upper body relaxed and moving easily. If you hold your hands in fists, your entire arm, neck, and even face, will tense up, causing running to be more strenuous and less efficient. And, as many of us hold stress in our jaws and shoulders, it is important to learn to release the tension in these areas.

My first running coach told me to imagine holding a potato chip between my thumb and index finger, where the goal is to get through the run without breaking, or dropping the imaginary chip. He told me that if I could keep my hands relaxed, my arms would relax too, giving way to my shoulders and jaw. And he was right. By relaxing my hands, I could create a domino effect that helped my whole upper body to soften and let go.

I usually picture a Pringles chip, because those suckers are pretty darn easy to break. Trying to get through even a thirty minute run without breaking (or dropping) the imaginary chip takes deliberate relaxation, and that is what we'll be doing with today's mudra exercise.

Belly Breathing

The mudra for connectivity takes this common runner's exercise one step further. I recently heard Deepak Chopra say that holding fists creates a shallow, chest breathing pattern, while practicing this mudra (index finger to thumb) promotes rhythmic, diaphragmatic breathing, or what is referred to as "belly breath" in yoga. Belly breathing increases your sense of calm and overall well being, by filling your lungs fully, slowing down your rate of respiration, and helping you to relax. As your lungs fully inflate, they send rich, oxygenated blood out to the rest of the body, whereby the tissues are nourished. As the body receives this rich, oxygenated breath, it relaxes. It releases tension. It lets go. As this happens, you feel better.

You may notice that, initially, you will feel like slowing your pace a bit, as simply touching your fingers together and relaxing your hand promotes a sense of ease, and flow. But as your run progresses, you'll notice how this ease and flow actually work to your benefit. Filling your lungs completely with diaphragmatic breath, nourishing the body's tissues with oxygenated blood, and holding the hands, arms, face, and jaw relaxed, not only helps you to feel better, it helps you to run more efficiently, which translates to faster and longer.

And, the yogis believe that the connectivity mudra increases our connection to God, all that is, the Universe, the Collective Consciousness, the Soul, the Highest Self...whatever you call it, it reminds us that we are not alone. Placing your index finger and thumb gently together creates a gesture of union.

Today's Run

So do it today. Carry this beneficial mudra with you out on your run. Remember that by gently touching your index finger and thumb together, you'll be reducing your stress levels by promoting belly breathing. You'll run in a more relaxed and efficient manner because your arms, neck, and face will be relaxed, and you'll be reminded that you are connected to, and guided by, something greater than yourself.

Now, get your mudra on, and go run yourself happy today! And by all means, don't stop with your run. Take this simple relaxation technique out with you into the world. Anytime you feel stressed or overwhelmed, gently hold your hands in this mudra for connectivity. You'll trigger a chain reaction of relaxation, and be reminded that you are connected to all that is. You are guided.

Post-Run Journal:

Today's Run Yourself Happy task was subtle and deliberate. Did you notice a shift? What did you notice on your run today?

CHEST ALIVE

Here's a great one for you! The purpose of today's Chest Alive practice is to help you to get out of your head, and into your body. You'll breathe away worry, and cultivate calm, ease, and joy.

Take a minute before you start your run to get a few deep breaths in through your nose and out through your nose or mouth. Slow yourself down a bit, and let your body relax.

Now close your eyes and continue breathing this way, but visualize a giant nose right in the middle of your chest, on your heart chakra. Yes, I said a "giant nose." You know, like the ones that come with plastic "disguise" glasses. You can even give it a mustache if you'd like. Below your imaginary nose, where your diaphragm is, picture a smile line. A simple, smiley face, like the ones you drew on notes to your friends, before we texted everything and used emoticons. :)

Imagine, that as you breathe in, breath is going in through those giant nostrils, right there on your chest. You are breathing into your heart chakra. The heart chakra is the body's energy center for love, balance, and compassion. For me, the heart chakra is also a place where I hold my deepest, most vulnerable fears.

The desires of our heart are the desires of the soul, and are therefore, incredibly vulnerable. Breathing into the heart chakra is important to open up to love and release fear. It is imperative

59

if you wish to follow your heart and live in the space of your soul's calling. Make no mistake, living in your soul's calling is an essential component of a happy and fulfilling life.

Heart Nose

Now, as you go out on your run, you don't have to actually try to breathe through your chest... but as you run today, continue to *imagine* that the big nose on your chest is breathing straight into your heart; making room for love, compassion, and forgiveness. Be prepared, this simple idea of breathing into that giant nose on your chest may evoke an emotional response that you are not expecting. There's beauty in being on a run while it happens. Just allow it. Keep breathing, and keep running, but allow yourself to feel, and to release. Go ahead and snot rocket if you have to.

Diaphragm Smile

The smile on your diaphragm reminds you to breathe in joy, and release everything else. It also happens to be located near your third chakra, the solar plexus. This is where I tend to hold my anxiety. The solar plexus is your place of personal power, self esteem, and warrior energy. It is also where "gut feelings" come from. Placing an imaginary smile here, while you breathe in love and release fear and negativity, is a reminder to smile at yourself. Be joyful. Know that you are safe and supported.

As you breathe into the giant nose on your heart chakra, you might experience some emotions that are uncomfortable, but the smile on your diaphragm will be there to remind you that it is all ok. The simple imaginary smile will be a friend, offering love and support, as you breathe through whatever emotions come up.

Question for the Day

As you are breathing into your heart and smiling in your power center, you may choose to pose a question to your subconscious. "How can I follow my heart today?" Don't feel pressure to answer this question. Just keep it in your consciousness, and return to the image of the nose on your heart, and the smile on your diaphragm. As you run, keep today's question in mind, and carry it with you into your day. How can you follow your heart today? Let that great big, imaginary nose do all of the work today, and smile into the knowing that this exercise, silly as it may seem, actually works wonders.

That's it! Go run with a big chest nose and a diaphragm smile. I promise, you will come back feeling refreshed, rejuvenated, and well...happier! Happiness isn't reached in one fell swoop, or with one great achievement. Happiness is derived from the small choices we make every day to answer the call of our soul.

Post Run Journal

What came up for you on the run today? How did you feel physically? Emotionally?

HORSE, DUCK, DOG

WARNING: People may look at you funny today!

Today's run is going to be awesome, because you'll be releasing old patterns that keep you stuck in a negative stress response, and making way for clean, calm, new energy! Plus, you will have to laugh at yourself because you'll be jiggling, shaking, and flapping all over the place! It's the most "active" practice of the week, and it has several components. You can choose to use them all today, or spread them out over the next few days. I recommend the latter if you are new to this stuff.

Horse Lips

I learned about horse lips from a high school teammate, and all-around stud-runner named Shelley Taylor. Shelly had these amazing Angelina Jolie lips, so it made the demonstration awesome! And, because she was kind of a big deal in high school running at the time, I took this little suggestion to heart, and still use it today.

Shelley told me to do this exercise as a way to slow down my breathing. I used to see her do it as a way to slow down and relax her breathing and body between hard intervals. Usually, she would accompany the horse lips with some arm and hand shaking. It was pretty silly looking... but she was older and faster than me, so I did it too.

Here's What to Do:

Try it now, while you read this. Relax your face, cheeks, and jaw. Gently close your mouth and lips. Not tightly sealed, just relaxed and shut. Inhale deeply through your nose, and exhale deeply (and somewhat forcefully) through your closed lips. You should make a bilabial "pbpbpbpb" sound, and if you do it right, your lips will flap around like a horse's. You may even fling spit! Another way to imagine this is making the motor boat in the bathtub noise. Remember that? Putting your face halfway underwater and turning your lips into the engine? Same thing!

It might be hard, at first, to produce the horse lips sound. Especially if you are really pissed off. All that means is that you are holding too much tension in your face. Just keep taking slow, relaxed breaths, while deliberately relaxing your face, lips, and jaw. It may be helpful (and fun!) to add the motorboat sound to it.

Here's Why You Do It:

Shelley Taylor was absolutely right! As it turns out, taking time to deliberately slow your exhale is a powerful tool for relaxation. Creating the horse lips is nearly impossible if your face and jaw are tense, and to really get the effect to last, you'll need to cultivate a diaphragmatic breath. Shaking out the shoulders, arms, and hands, simultaneously just adds to the release of tension.

Duck Flap

I am reminded of a video I once saw about the importance of physically "shaking off" negative energy. Humans have an unfortunate habit of holding on to negative experiences, and continually replaying them in our heads, and holding them in our bodies. When we replay a negative scenario in our heads, we actually replay our body's physiological response as well. More times than not, the physiological response to a negative experience is a stress response. It triggers the release of stress hormones, and causes that familiar pang if anxiety, worry, sadness, anger, or what-have-you. So, by re-telling the "Oh-my-GOD-you-are-not-going-to *believe*-this," story of how you were wronged, to friends, or even just thinking about it on a run, you literally create more stress and unhappiness in your body.

Ducks are different. The video I mention was about ducks. I recall that it showed two ducks fighting. There was angry quacking, flapping, and some pecking as well. When the fight was over, though, each of the respective ducks flew off to separate areas of the pond, landed, and had themselves a good wing-flapping shake. Then, they relaxed into the peace and ease of being a duck, without having to quack on and on about the injustice of it to all of their friends. They didn't have to re-tell the story, or re-live the ways in which they had been wronged. They glided peacefully on the placid pond of life, free from any residual anger and stress.

Shelley used to flap out the tension while running, and as I learned to mimic her, I felt the results for myself. Letting go of the tension I carried in my arms, by simply letting them dangle and flap from my shoulders as I ran for a few steps, was extremely rejuvenating. I found that I did feel better, and was able to run with much more ease as I picked my arms back up again.

Wet Dog Shake

How many times do we hear it on the athletic field? "Just shake it off." But what if it really works? What if literally shaking your body like a dog out of a bath, actually *does* release stress, tension, and negativity? Try it right now. Stand up and give your body a good shake. Seriously, right now. Put the book down, and try it. Imagine the head to toe wiggle a dog does after a bath, and give it a go. I'll wait....

Doesn't that feel better? Silly, but better, right?!?!

The Importance of Silliness

As it turns out, silliness is a seriously important part of our happiness practice. Silliness isn't necessarily attached to results, but, it naturally elicits joy. While we do have an agenda of relaxation and release with today's shake and flap running, the silliness factor is undeniable. You *will* look silly, which means that you must be willing to *be* silly.

So do it! Take it to the next level. Pretend to be a horseduckdog. Make silly noises. Exaggerate your movements. Enjoy your own brand of crazy, and just go with it. Life is too short to judge yourself for how you look while running! And, no offense, but I am betting there are plenty of times that you've looked pretty silly on a run without even trying to. Remember that outfit from last week? Or when you ate crap in a fantastic trip over a tree root? At least for today, embrace it. We don't have to take ourselves so seriously.

On Your Run Today:

Today, on your run, you will need to channel your inner duck, dog, and horse! Is there something that habitually bothers you? Maybe someone who continually rubs you the wrong way? An ex-boyfriend or girlfriend? A mother-in-law? That guy who sits at the cubicle across from you? Or a situation where you felt truly wronged or betrayed? When you go running with a negative a situation that causes you to feel resentful, you also bring your body's stress response. What you think about on your runs affects your body.

What you can do today, to release and relax, is breathe like a horse, flap like a duck, and shake like a dog! Every time you catch your mind telling the old negative story that get's your blood boiling again, *do* it! You don't have to stop running, but shake, flap, and do the horse lips! If you can simultaneously tell yourself, "I choose to release this situation" while doing it, you get bonus points. But, just the physical movements will lift your heart, lighten your mood, release tension and cultivate calm.

You may get some interesting looks, but you'll be so happy that you just won't care!

Post Run Journal

How did it feel to look silly today? What physical sensations did you experience before, during, and after, your run?

Chapter 10
WEEK 2

Ignite Imagination

In chapter nine, you learned three techniques to help release stress from the body. These may seem and feel silly, but as you have experienced by now, they really do work. This week, you can continue to use the techniques you learned in chapter nine. Hopefully they will become automatic soon, but we're also going to add another layer to your Run Yourself Happy practice. This week is about the power of imagination.

Imagination is the single most powerful tool that humans possess. And yet, by the time we are in the third or fourth grade, much of it is lost. I don't generally like to get up on a negative soap box, but I passionately believe that the current system of education in the United States is literally sucking the creative juices, and more importantly, the confidence, out of most of the children it is meant to serve.

I was a very bright and imaginative student, and school was actually quite easy for me. I was eager to learn and participate, and, since I enjoyed writing, I excelled. But the problem was that I was looking for the "right answer." Ultimately, my success in school was directly related, not to the quality and imaginative nature of my thoughts, but to my ability to please my teachers with the responses that they were hoping for.

While I have no idea whether or not you were successful in school, it is likely that some element of my story resonates with you, because, if you grew up in the United States, this is the social conditioning you received. There are right answers and wrong ones. There is the correct interpretation of a story, and an incorrect, or misguided one. We've learned to stop thinking outside of the box and start looking for the right answers.

The problem with this is that it stops us from considering possibilities. It inhibits our imaginations. When we believe that there is a right answer, we also tend to believe that there is a particular way to arrive at that answer. We accept what we have been taught. We're told that the teacher is right, and in many cases, punished if we question his or her authority.

And we may have been parented this way as well. My parents loved me very much, and they truly wanted the best for me, but they inadvertently taught me not to follow my dreams. They had an idea that the best course for me would be to become educated, get a secure job (teacher or nurse were strongly encouraged), marry a hardworking and stable man, and live happily ever after.

But I wanted to be a star! I wanted to be on television, or be a supermodel, or a world famous author. While they never told me that these were impossible dreams, they may as well have, because they didn't tell me to pursue them with all of my heart. They told me the statistics; that it was very unlikely that I would "make it" at these professions, and that I had better have a safe and reliable back up plan.

I don't blame them for this. I understand that it came from their own fears. But I do acknowledge that this conditioning isn't truth.

The truth is that we are put on this earth to live out our soul's calling. We are born with innate gifts and desires that ought to be nurtured and protected, rather than dismissed and discouraged. And, if the light inside of us is a mere smolder in the ashes of a burning desire that is all but extinguished, it is our responsibility to rekindle the fire. Our life's purpose is to live the life that lights us up inside.

I'm reminded of the famous Marianne Williamson quote:

> *"Our deepest fear is not that we are inadequate. Our deepest fear is that we are powerful beyond measure. It is our light, not our darkness that most frightens us. We ask ourselves, Who am I to be brilliant, gorgeous, talented, fabulous? Actually, who are you not to be? You are a child of God. Your playing small does not serve the world. There is nothing enlightened about shrinking so that other people won't feel insecure around you. We are all meant to shine, as children do. We were born to make manifest the glory of God that is within us. It's not just in some of us; it's in everyone.*

And as we let our own light shine, we unconsciously give other people permission to do the same. As we are liberated from our own fear, our presence automatically liberates others."

In this chapter you will be using your imagination to blow on the ashes and reignite the flame of the light inside of you. You will be running with the intention to re-birth old dreams and give birth to new ones. You will speak your dreams and desires into reality, and create a community of loving and supportive trees (yes, I said *trees*). And, you will be connecting lovingly to your body, after releasing fear.

Each of this week's Run Yourself Happy practices will connect you more deeply with the little girl in you with big dreams. You will be lovingly reprogramming your subconscious and connecting with your higher self as you go. Get ready! This week's work is transformative.

As with each week of the program, please continue to do your alignment practices and run with a friend at least once a week. You'll need the support from your skeletal structure as well as your running buddy.

DREAMRUNNING

Dreamrunning is a favorite running pastime, and one that really gets me in the mood to create a magnificent life. And don't worry, you'll be fully awake!

It requires very little mental discipline and is a whole lot of fun to do.

Did you know that day-dreaming is actually a productive pastime? Yes. Dreaming about what you would like to achieve in your life, and enjoying the feelings that these dreams evoke, actually helps to *create* (ie: manifest) your dreams.

Your imagination is the most powerful tool you have, not only in releasing stress and tension (as we played with last chapter), but in creating the life that you desire. Albert Einstein said, "Imagination is more powerful than knowledge," and just for today, let's assume that he was right. Let's assume that the ability to *imagine* your full-blown miracle life is more powerful than *knowing* how to get it.

Be a Dreamer

My husband calls me a "Dreamer." And, truth be told, this often sounds more like an accusation, than a compliment. It makes me sad, because I know that dreaming is such an important skill. That's right, I said *skill*. You see, we are all born dreamers.

Children have incredible imaginations and can dream just about anything into reality. They are powerful manifesters. But as we get older, we have our dreams squeezed out of us. We're told to "be realistic." We're taught that happiness fits into a pretty box with a college degree and a six figure salary. We're put on a track for success and happiness that may have very little to do with our dreams, or our soul's purpose.

At the same time, we're force-fed subjects in school that may have little or no relevance to the life we wish to create. We're told to "stop daydreaming and pay attention." But we need to pay attention to our daydreams. We must listen to our inner desires, no matter how "unrealistic" they may seem. Our soul speaks to us in daydreams. They feel good because they are right for us. In order to be happy adults, we must re-learn how to dream. We must allow ourselves to believe in our dreams, and this is a skill that may take a little practice.

For now, don't worry about how completely impossible it may seem to get from where you currently are, to the life that you dream of. Just allow yourself to dream, and pay attention to any emergent themes.

Some Dream Starters

When I win the lottery....

When I was little, I wanted to...

If money wasn't a concern, I would...

If I knew I wouldn't fail, I would...

If I wasn't so afraid, I'd....

My favorite dream starter is the lottery win, because I actually do plan on winning the Mega Millions or Powerball jackpots. But, more importantly, it helps me to get clear about what really matters to me, and the direction I would like to lean in my life. I think about what my daily life will be like after I win the lottery. What types of things will I do with my time? Where will I live? Would I move at all? What kinds of people will I be spending my time with? What will some of my big purchases be? What will I choose to do with all of my wealth? How will I serve the world? What will I *create* when lack of money is no longer an issue?

As I get clear, I can turn some of these dreams into goals. Or, I can just continue to fantasize about them. Either way, I'll be more aware of what I'd like my life to be like.

Prophetic Daydreams

What used to continually come up for me in my lottery life vision, is that I would like to run in beautiful places, and life coach motivated clients while I ran. I also saw myself as an author, whose work made a big impact, and a seminar leader and inspirational speaker. Then, I saw myself creating this book, and creating a Run Yourself Happy movement. I began to see possibility after possibility, and it all felt like a pretty awesome way to spend my time.

Since, in my vision, I'd already won the lottery, this work was a reward within itself. This is important to recognize, because these things are clearly my soul's work. Why else would they be so important for me to do *after* I win the lottery? And guess what?!? After spending time on my runs, literally letting my imagination "run free" with this idea, some pretty incredible synchronicities occurred that allowed this dream to begin to unfold.

One Caveat

Once you have energetically charged your dreams, you must obey the guidance that comes to you. My little reminder slogan is: *move daily in the direction of your dreams.*

Start a vision board. Join a group of like-minded people. Invest in the Run Yourself Happy System (http://runyourselfhappysystem.com), or just journal about it. But take action, no matter how small it may seem, in the direction of your dreams. Little energetic offerings amount to major shifts over time. The more you vibrate at the frequency of your dreams, the more you will be attracting them to you.

So Get Going

Lace those shoes up and get your dream on! Today's run is all about daydreaming. Let your imagination run wild, and imagine what you want your life to be like. Use my dream starters (see questions above) if you find them helpful, and get running. Dreamrunning is good for the soul, so go do it!

Post Run Journal:

Write about your dreams. Use a dream starter and let your imagination run wild.

TALK TO THE TREES

Today's Run Yourself Happy exercise will help you to feel connected and supported. It's awesome; and it's one of my favorites.

Yes, you read the heading correctly. Today you will be talking to the trees. I actually stole this idea from Pam Grout who wrote about using this technique in E^2: *nine do it yourself energy experiments that prove your thoughts create your reality.* As I have mentioned, using the techniques in this book seemed to come very naturally on my daily runs, and was a catalyst for my deciding to write this book. This particular technique is my absolute favorite for creating a feeling of connectedness and support.

So, here's the gist. Today, on your run, you are going to talk to the trees. Sound crazy? Just bear with me. In my years of personal growth and development, as well as my study of the Law of Attraction, I've found a common thread. If you want something to happen, you must *believe* it is going to happen. You must act as if it has already happened. Your cells must be vibrating at the frequency of whatever it is you hope to attract. So, if you wish to attract a million dollars, you need to feel, inside, that you already have that million dollars. You must vibrate wealth in order to attract wealth. This used to be a catch twenty-two for me, until I started talking to the trees.

You see, if you come from a place of needing a million dollars, you are attracting the *need* of that million dollars, and therefore will attract more need, rather than the actual million bucks. And, while "acting as if" is a good idea, it doesn't work if you can't *feel* it. The same goes for "putting it out there." Talking about how you are going to manifest a million dollars, or your soul mate, or a new car, or whatever it is you desire, only "puts out" the energy that you genuinely feel behind your goal.

In the past, I have told people plenty of times that I am writing a book, and I have literally started dozens of them, but the energy behind wanting to write these books was about desperation. It was about *wanting* to write a book. I didn't feel worthy, valuable, or qualified enough to actually be a successful author. I was afraid that I didn't have what it takes to finish, or that I didn't have anything of value to say. No amount of talking about the books that I was writing could trick the Universe into believing me, because *I* didn't believe me. My vibrations didn't lie. Emit desperation, get back more desperation.

But, like I said, all of this changed when I started talking to the trees. Here is why. Trees are living, breathing organisms. They have their own energetic fields, just like you and me. And, also like us, they are receptive to the energetic fields of others. In other words, trees can feel our energy.

The awesome thing about trees is that they literally breathe in our breath and exhale it back out to us in the form of oxygen. Trees are connected to heaven and earth. They breathe "the breath of life" out into the heavens, but they are "rooted" in the earth. I love the image of the roots... like a secret underground network.

This is what I do:

I tell a tree something that I want to manifest. It might be a career goal. It might be something that I am working on personally. I might tell the trees that I am willing to forgive someone, or that I'm willing to feel safe and loved. The important thing is that it is something that I really want to be true, and that I just need a little help believing.

I say it out loud to the first few trees that I pass, and I ask them to pass it on. I imagine that the trees are taking my intentions and broadcasting them to the Universe. I imagine them breathing my wishes into the atmosphere, and sending them in messages on their leaves. I see my intentions broadcast through the root network, and spreading to the water supply, the Earth, and the animals that inhabit it. I feel my intentions being honored by the trees, and imagine that they are excited to help me.

Before long, I am feeling grateful, confident, and supported. I totally believe whatever it is that I've been telling the trees, and I am getting pretty excited about it. I begin to touch the trees as I tell them my intentions and sense them encouraging me. Soon, I notice branches and vines reaching out to me as I run, and I "high five" them as I go, feeling victorious. I finish my run in a very different energetic space than I started, and can now act and speak with confidence about whatever it is I intend to manifest, because I know that my intentions have been energetically broadcast across the tree network.

Just Try it!

Don't worry about appearing crazy (hopefully you're getting used to it by now)! Just try it. When you are on your run today, imagine that as you talk to a tree, it spreads the word through its secret root network, by exhaling it to the heavens, and sending messages on the leaves blowing in the wind. Hear the rustle of the leaves and know that it is the trees sending your message. Imagine, that as you tell a tree what you want, the tree passes it on to the next tree, and the next. Know that you are loved and supported by the trees that you pass on your run.

The Rules of Tree Talking:

Be positive. Be sure to tell the trees what you want in the form of an affirmation. If you just can't feel genuine in affirming something that isn't currently true, try using the phrase "I'm willing to" or "I'm ready to." One that I have been saying lately is "I earn my first two million dollars within the next two years. Pass it on." Notice that I am not reinforcing my *want* of the two million dollars, but the fact that I earn it.

To be clear, when I started telling the trees this idea, I had absolutely no idea of how I could possibly earn two million dollars over the next two years, but after using it for a while, the "how" has started to unfold in truly miraculous ways. I absolutely know that if I had started speaking this affirmation to people, I would have felt awkward and ingenuine. Saying it out loud would have given rise to my fears, doubts, and insecurities. That's why I started with the trees. They are an easy place to feel God's presence. There's just something magical about trees.

Start Today

Get out there, and talk to the trees today. Smile at them. Thank them for supporting you. Give them high fives. Sure, passerbys may think you've lost it, but you will have shifted your energy and you'll feel the magic of this incredibly responsive Universe! You'll be happier because you'll feel connected to the powerful Source Energy, Higher Power, God, the Universe...whatever you choose to call it; that connects us all.

Start small if you'd like. Tell the trees that you expect to see a tiger in the next 24 hours. Then, when the tiger shows up (in real life, on a book cover, an internet video, a stuffed toy, or another form), you'll have the solid proof you need to continue talking to the trees.

PS.

Of all of the Run Yourself Happy exercises in this book, this one is my favorite. I use it at least once a week, still. I absolutely know that talking to the trees is a major reason for the miraculous shift that has occurred in my life, and I am so grateful to have discovered it.

Post Run Journal

What did you say to the trees today? How did it feel? What insights came to you as you ran?

TALK TO YOUR BODY WITH LOVE

I absolutely believe that we can heal ourselves with the power of our thoughts. The work of people like Dr. Bruce Lipton and Dr. Masaru Emoto have shown us that the energy that surrounds a cell or molecule of water can literally change the structure of that cell or molecule.

Dr. Emoto is famous for his experiments with water crystals, showing us that when we send the water positive energy in the form of soothing music, positive words, and even beautiful photographs, it reacts by forming beautiful crystals. But negative words and angry music produce irregular and misshapen crystals. Same water; different energy around them. What he noticed was that the molecules rearranged themselves based on the *energy* of the words, music, or photos. In other words, positive messages yielded beautiful crystal, while negative messages yielded ugly ones.

The same is true of our cells. Dr Bruce Lipton, author of *The Biology of Belief* shows us that it is not the nucleus of the cell that determines the cell's health and activity, but rather the energetic environment of the cell. Just like water crystals, our cells react favorably or unfavorably to the energy we send them. Positive energy yields positive results. Since our bodies are made up largely of water, this is not surprising.

Marinate on that

Now, I'd like you to take a moment to really allow that to sink in. If this is the first time you have digested information like this, it can be a little mind blowing. What I am saying is that every cell in your body reacts to the messages that they receive. Cells receive messages in the form of energy. Sound energy, light energy, emotional energy, thought energy...it's all *vibrational* in nature. Put simply, your body vibrates to the tune that you play to it. It will change over time to reflect what you think about it, and what you choose to believe about it. If you constantly expose your body to negativity, it will react negatively.

So take a minute to think about the messages you inadvertently send your cells all day, every day. Do you say things like "I'm fat," "I'm slow," "I'm tired," "I'm sore," "I'm sick," etc? And could changing your inner vocabulary *really* change your body on a molecular level?

Really? I Mean, Really?

Absolutely! Now, does this mean that if you have a stress fracture and you go running while chanting to yourself "my bones are strong and healthy," that you will come back miraculously healed? While I never discount the possibility of a miracle when it is backed by a strong belief, I will say that these types of changes generally take time. This is because the power to change the molecules lies in the energy that surrounds them, and while words carry a powerful energy, so does subconscious belief. If you go on a run saying to yourself, "I'm lean and fit," but you have a subconscious belief that you will always struggle with your weight, then the belief will likely win out. This is because the power of feelings is very strong, and quite frankly, your subconscious runs your life.

Your Subconscious Beliefs

The thing about subconscious beliefs is that they are below the level of consciousness (duh! Hence the name, sub-conscious). In other words, you have beliefs that you don't even recognize. These beliefs are formed very early in our lives, and generally come from conclusions we drew as children. For instance, if you were criticized as a child, you may likely have a belief that you'll never be good enough. And, while you may have done plenty of work to convince yourself that you are awesome and worthy of the very best that life has to offer, if you do not see that evidenced in your life and often feel that no matter what you do, it's still not good enough, it is because you're still carrying around the negative subconscious belief.

So how do you change them? There are several layers to this, and you could fill entire bookstores on the research and methodologies around changing subconscious beliefs. But don't let any of that scare you. Just be open to the possibility that they can be changed. Accept the possibility that, by changing your subconscious "operating system," you can completely shift your outer reality.

And let's keep it simple. You can begin to change your subconscious beliefs by telling yourself a new story, and infusing that story with the *feeling* that you intend to create. Today's run will be focused on talking to your cells, and telling them a new story.

On Your Run

For today, I'd like you to talk lovingly to your cells. Think of yourself as the Divine Parent to each and every little baby cell in your amazing body. Imagine that your voice is the voice of God to your cells. As you run today, talk to your body with love. Be grateful, proud, and encouraging. And speak miracles into reality.

For example, if you are frustrated with the extra layer of fat that you are carrying around your mid-section, try speaking something like this to your body while focusing your mind and imagination on your midsection:

> *Hello sweet cells. Thank you so much for being such incredibly obedient little children. I have sent you messages of fear and worry, and you have responded by creating fat cells that insulate me from the world. Thank you so much for wanting to protect me. But I am ready to let go. My sweet cells, it is time for us to release all of that fear and insulation, and shine in all of our beauty and brilliance. [Imagine your cells' response. See them in your mind's eye, and feel the love that they feel.]*

> *Beautiful body, you are an incredible creation. You are meant to radiate perfect health and balance. You are lean, fit, and totally beautiful, and I lovingly give you permission to show this. I love you and I enjoy running with you. Fat cells, I ask that you burn off the extra energy that you are holding. I no longer need it to keep me safe. I love you. [Imagine the fat cells shrinking as they release fear and radiate love.]*

Or maybe you are struggling with and illness or injury. The same basics apply. Send love to your body. Commend it for being so responsive and obedient to you. After all, if you have an injury or illness, your thoughts have played a very large part in creating it. So, do your part in healing it. Send that injury love and release it.

Thank your illness for coming into to your life, acknowledge your part in creating it, then bless it and send it on its way. Ask your cells to rearrange themselves into their intended state of perfect health. By sending love to your cells and reframing the story you tell yourself, you will be making subtle shifts in your subconscious. The more you do this, the more powerful the change will be.

Miracles happen when you move from fear to love. So, no matter what the story in your mind is, see if you can find the role of fear and infuse the story with love.

What to Expect

It is important to say that this activity will be much more powerful if you are able to actually speak the words out loud while you run. This is true for two reasons. The first is that your mind is less likely to wander off if you are speaking out loud to yourself rather than just in your head. And the second is that words really do have power over the molecules in our bodies. As we speak, so it is. Speaking lovingly to your body will be powerful.

About that. Like many of the activities I ask you to do in this book, it is likely that you will have an unexpected emotional response. As always, just allow and honor that. Today's activity asks you to speak to your body as you would, ideally, speak to a child that you love unconditionally. You will be speaking to your body what your subconscious needs to hear, and likely, didn't from your parents. Honor that. Flood your cells with love and acceptance, and allow them to release the subconscious negativity that you've carried around for years.

Just Do It

So get out there and run. Speak lovingly to your body and focus on the places in your body that you generally resent or chastise. Imagine that the cells there are your sweet babies. Acknowledge your part in creating the undesirable condition, and empower your cells to change. Little by little, the miracle will occur. Heal your thoughts, and you will heal your body.

Post-Run Journal

What did you experience on your run today? If you felt resistance to your new story, what was it? Bless the resistance and forgive yourself. You may want to write a letter of love and acceptance to your three to six year old self.

Chapter 11
WEEK 3

Invite Intuition

Last week, you got busy with your imagination. Some of the exercises may have pushed you out of your comfort zone a bit, but hopefully you found them fun and beneficial. So, you've learned techniques for releasing bodily stress and accessing the power of your imagination. Please continue to practice them as you see fit this week. However, we'll also be adding another layer. This week is all about inviting and accessing your intuition.

I love week three! I love it because intuition is such an amazing gift that we all have. I love it because inviting intuition into your life is so incredibly freeing. I love it because nurturing and listening to my intuition has made all of the difference in my life. Following my intuition has absolutely been the key to my currently happy, and generally anxiety-free, existence.

If you are wondering what, exactly, intuition is, allow me to explain. Intuition is that "still small voice" or "gut feeling" that guides you. Have you ever met someone and just known that you'd be friends? You just "had a feeling?" That is intuition. It is the wiser, broader part of you that is connected to the mysterious fabric of the Universe.

I don't mean to get all cryptic here, but tapping into your intuition in pretty darn magical! And, if you listen to it, it can be an infallible guidance system. In this chapter, you'll let your intuition be your guide. You'll learn to use the sensations in your body to "tune in" to your intuitive knowings.

The Gifts of Intuition

One of the gifts of my intuitive voice is that it's persistent. And it tends to speak to me on my runs. It's not like I hear a booming: "This is your Intuition Speaking" type of announcement, but it speaks to me in the form of recurring thoughts, daydreams, and ideas that just feel right. I might have a thought like, "I need to call Jamie." If this is the voice of my intuition, and I choose not to act on it, reasons to call Jamie will continue to show up in my life until I actually pick up the phone and call her. I may see something that reminds me of her. I might get an email from her, or my husband might randomly ask me about her. The point is: if I have an intuitive knowing that I need to call her, I'll get plenty of reminders.

I love the way Oprah Winfrey talks about intuition. She says that it starts talking to you in whispers, and if you ignore them, it will tap you on the shoulder. If you ignore that, your intuition will give you a nudge, and then a shove. If you ignore those, you'll get pushed into a brick wall! This push into a brick wall looks and feels like a disaster in your life. It is your soul's way of letting you know that you are not on the right track, and is an opportunity to change.

Intuition is persistent for a reason. It has your best interest in mind, and its job is to help guide you on the path to living your life's purpose. The job of your intuition is to be your internal guidance system. It's like the GPS of your soul.

Another gift of intuition is that it is experiential. You can feel it in your body. It's quite primal, actually. It's easy to recognize once you know how.

How to Listen to Intuition

The trick to listening to your intuition is not second guessing yourself. Don't try to rationalize, just act in good faith. Once, when I was in high school, I was running down a car lined street on my way back to school from the beach. I saw a man standing between two cars and instantly felt an "inner ding" that something about this man was "off." But the next thing that came into my head was my mother's voice saying, "Now Carrie, don't judge." And then my rational mind went to work. This street was full of cars because many beach-goers didn't want to pay for parking. It was a popular spot for surfers to park and walk to the beach. For this reason, it was not uncommon to see men between cars or behind car doors, with towels wrapped around their waists, shimmying in and out of wetsuits.

However, as I approached this particular man, I still couldn't shake the feeling that he should be avoided. Not wanting to offend him, however, I proceeded. And, as I reached the front of the car that he was standing behind, he stepped out into plain view, naked from the waist down, with the clear intention of displaying himself to me.

At sixteen, this was both shocking and terrifying, but I am lucky that he was "just a flasher." I am grateful that his intention was merely to shock me, and not to attack. My intuition gave me all the signals, but I chose to second guess.

And the same is true for a positive "intuitive hit." When you get an intuitive knowing, follow it. It is in following our intuition that we create the space in our lives for the truly miraculous to occur. It will absolutely take you where you need to go. It may tell you something that doesn't make rational sense, but the more you learn to trust it, the more it will serve you.

This Week

In this chapter you'll use your daily run to invite intuition. By now, you may actually already feel more connected to the intuitive side of yourself. After all, you've been releasing stress and igniting your imagination; the path to hear the voice of your intuition has been cleared.

The Run Yourself Happy practices offered this week are intended to help bridge the gap between the you that is your personality, and the You that is connected to all that is.

As always, continue to layer the practices from the weeks prior whenever it feels right. You'll know what to do when. Trust yourself. And please don't forget your alignment and run with a friend practices. They are so important to keeping yourself on track.

Alright, get out there, and enjoy your runs this week!

RUN WATCHLESS

Today's Run Yourself Happy practice is designed to remind you that no matter how you may be feeling at the moment, you are guided, and you are in exactly the space you need to be, to learn what you need to learn, and grow in the ways that you need to grow.

This can be a bit uncomfortable to recognize and accept if you find yourself feeling dissatisfied and unhappy with your life circumstances. Perhaps you are pushing hard in a particular area of your life, and finding yourself facing one roadblock and struggle after another.

Often times, when we find ourselves in this type of situation, it is because we are either on the wrong path, or we are on the right path, but we have allowed our ego to be in control. We have forgotten to surrender.

The ego's main job is to try to convince you that it *is* you. But you are not your ego. No matter what your religious beliefs, try to wrap your head around that fact that you are a "child of God," "a Divine Creation," and are more than just the sum of your parts. You have a soul, which is the broader, wiser, more connected part of your being, and this, my friend, is who you really are. You are neither your ego, nor your body. You are Divine, my dear. You are an energetic force. You absolutely *are* what you want to become.

But, in order to get into alignment with the You that is far greater than your ego or your body, you absolutely must be willing to listen to that greater part of yourself. You must be willing to set aside your plans, and follow the guidance that comes your way.

Leave Your Watch (or GPS, or Phone) at Home

As I employ this strategy more and more on my daily runs, I am amazed by the results. Running without a watch has been a huge metaphor in my life. And, I notice that I get injured less, feel better when I run, and look forward to running for the pure joy of doing it. I am reminded of the many ways in my life I hold on to the illusion of control.

The Illusion of Control

Control is an illusion. It's a lie we tell ourselves. It is not real. Control is a myth. And believing in control cannot lead to true happiness. Not the kind of joyful, whole hearted, full-blown miracle existence that you are seeking. I know that is hard to swallow, especially if you hold a belief that you will be happy when everything in your environment is just right. It was hard for me too. While I like to blame all of the "control issues" in my household on my husband, it's fair to say that I can be a control freak too. But what I need to remember is that believing in control is believing in my ego. And I am bigger, greater, and wiser than my ego. My ego thinks it knows the answers. It thinks it can control the outcomes of my actions. But my soul... my soul allows miracles.

Today's Metaphor

The watch and the workout plan are the control factor in today's running metaphor. The fear based belief is, that if you don't log the right amount of miles, at the right pace, then you ought to be disappointed in yourself, or feel guilty because you must do what the workout calendar says in order to achieve your goal. But your soul knows. Your soul is wiser, and already knows the outcome.

Listen to it. Allow yourself, your body, and your thoughts to be guided by a power greater than yourself. Have faith in your goals, and trust the wisdom of your inner guidance system to help you to reach them. Let go of the "way" that your ego sees. Just for today, let go of the "how." Open your heart and mind to the possibility that there you are guided. You are loved and supported by a force much greater than yourself, and it is conspiring on your behalf. Consider that by listening to your body, you are tuning in to one of the greatest communication devices of your soul. Today, you won't need your watch. You will let your intuition be your guide.

Panicking?

Just going running without a plan can actually be quite stressful for many of us control freaks. It can be downright terrifying to let go of our rigid beliefs about what we need to do in order to achieve our fitness goals, maintain our weight, or what have you. When I first attempted to "trust my body," I was bombarded with feelings of near panic. This just showed me how much my ego was in control. The ego rules by fear. So, the more you are afraid to do this activity, the more you need to. It can be terrifying. You may feel that if you dared to give your body control of the run, that it would totally slack. Heck, it might not even get out to door.

Here's what I have to offer about that. Think of your body as your teenage child that has just received his or her driver's license. On the one hand, you are terrified about all of the things that you, as the parent, cannot control. On the other hand, you know that if this child is to make it in the world, you will have to trust her to do the right things. You have an awareness that your child needs to learn to spread her wings. It is scary to hand over the keys. What about all of the other drivers on the road? Will she make wise decisions? What will she do with all of this newfound freedom? Will she make the choices that you want her to make? And there it is! Maybe she won't. Maybe she will make different choices, but if she is ever going to reach her true potential, she must make the choices herself. At some point, whether it is when she is sixteen, or heading off to college, you must hand over the keys.

Hand Over the Keys

And that is what you are going to do on today's run. You have been driving your body around for long enough. Trust that it knows your goals, and will make the right decisions to get you there. Trust that you are guided, not just toward your fitness goals, but *all* of your goals. Perhaps today's run will be a slight detour from what you had planned, but I promise that you will find yourself in exactly the right place, at exactly the right time.

Let your mind wander. Let your body do what it will. Run in peace, knowing that you don't need to do all of the driving. Your body and soul may take a slightly different route than you had planned, but they will not steer you wrong. You *will* get to your desired destination. So relax, and enjoy the ride. They may even take you to places you never dreamed you could go. Just hand over the keys.

Today's Run

So, for today, forget the run that you have planned. Today, you are going to listen to the broader, wiser part of you; your soul, your Higher Self, your Inner Guide. So, leave your watch at home. Let the wind take you where it will. Listen to your body, and to the call of your soul, and go running.

Allow yourself to be guided; to run without any idea of the pace you're running, or how many miles you are logging. Take a different route, and trust that it is the right one. Notice what you see. Notice where you are guided to go. Notice how you feel. Notice what you notice.

Maybe you will want to do some speed play, or run hills. Maybe you will want to run slower than you have ever allowed yourself to run before. Or faster. It doesn't really matter. Just do what feels right. Go where you feel the urge to go. It's ok. Trust that it is the right thing for you. It is. Allow yourself to feel great on your run today. Honor your body and allow it to do what it needs to do.

Post Run Journal

What insights came to you on your run today? What happened on your run? Pleasant surprises?

BODY AND SOUL

Today's practice involves a little bit of a mind tweak!

Your Body is an Antenna

Weird side note... did you know that when you are in a parking garage, looking for your car, and clicking the remote, hoping to hear the "beep," and see the lights flash, that the signal from the remote will actually go further if you hold it to your head? Your body is an antenna! It transmits and receives vibrational energy. Yep, it's a receiver for intuitive messages from your soul. You just need to be able to recognize the messages. And luckily, it's pretty easy once you know how! Messages from your soul feel great, empowering, peaceful, joyful, and all-around good.

But your body is also a transmitter. You are constantly vibrating messages out into the Universe. Have you ever walked into a room that felt heavy with grief? Even though no one said anything, you *felt* it when you walked in? That's because our bodies literally vibrate at the frequency of our thought and emotion. The bodies in the room are transmitting grief and your body acts as the receiver. Amazing, really!

Some of us believe that the soul is more of a concept than an actual thing. Others believe that it resides deep within the body. Others still, believe that the body lies within the energetic field of the soul.

These are interesting thoughts to ponder as you run today. What is your soul? How do you feel the call of *your* soul? Is there a part of the body that you associate with the soul?

I'm one of the people who tend to believe that the body resides within the soul. I like to imagine that my body lives within the "bubble of energetic light" that is my soul. I often close my eyes, and see my body surrounded by this white light. I feel guided, connected, and peaceful. I breathe deeply, and sometimes cry, but always feel love, encouragement, and a sense that all is well. I know that this feeling is an intuitive connection with my soul.

Good Vibes

When you feel good, energetic, inspired, etc.., it is because your current thoughts and actions are in alignment with your soul's calling; your higher purpose. In other words, you are on the right track. Your soul uses body sensations that feel good to communicate this to you. In this way, your body is the receiver.

Not-So-Good Vibes

When you are sick, injured, angry, anxious, or any other feeling in the body that doesn't feel good, this is your soul's gentle nudge that your current thoughts and actions are off track with your higher purpose. It is merely a reminder, from the part of you that is Love, that something is off.

A helpful affirmation when you are experiencing feelings or situations that are less than desirable is:

"I choose to see Love instead of this."

Just say it. Use it as a way to connect with your soul and ask for guidance.

Today's Run

As you run today, simply remind yourself that no matter what your ideas are about the soul, your experience of it occurs in your body. Your body is an instrument of your soul. It is a communication device between the "you" you identify as yourself, and your "Higher Self," or soul. Take these two affirmations with you as you pound the pavement or hit the trails today:

"I am not my body. I am the Force that animates it."

"My body is an instrument of my soul."

Just run with those, and see where they take you. Notice how you feel. As with many of the practices, it is not uncommon to feel highly emotional, angry, or uncomfortably vulnerable. Just accept what comes, and know that it is all part of the good work you are doing. You are re-connecting with the You you're meant to be. It's powerful work. Be gentle with yourself. And remember, you'll be happier for having done it.

Post Run Journal

What did you learn on your run today? What came up for you?

HAVE A CONVERSATION WITH GOD

Have you heard the old adage that the answers you seek are within you? Well, today you are going to learn how true this is. Today, you are going to have a conversation in your head, and the answers that you seek will be revealed.

I realize that is an incredibly bold claim. And today's Run Yourself Happy technique takes practice and patience, but, when you are able to get it, it will prove to be an incredibly powerful tool for self-discovery and personal growth. And, it will likely deepen your connection to whatever it is you call God.

Confession:

I often talk to myself when I run. I have full-on conversations in my head. I used to have these conversations with myself as a rehearsal for an upcoming conversation in my "real" life, or as a way to give myself a pep talk. And, while I still do those things occasionally, I have found the following technique to be downright awesome.

A Word on Words

For the purposes of this exercise, let's agree on a common vocabulary. When I refer to the *ego,* I'm talking about the voice in your head that you identify with you; your personality. This is the voice that chatters incessantly at you all day long, and if you've ever tried to meditate, it's the voice that you have trouble quieting. The voice of your ego is the voice of your thoughts. I often refer to this voice as "the bitch in my head," but for today, let's call it the ego.

I'm going to refer to the other voice as *God*. If it feels weird for you to think of it as God because you associate God with a bearded man on a cloud, or because you don't believe in God, or whatever, just select another word. Call it the Force, the Universe, the Divine, your Soul, or your Higher Self, or any of the other words I have already offered in this book. I often use these interchangeably because, quite frankly, the Wise Energy of All That Is, The ALL, is too massive to confine to one little word. So bear with me here. Hell, call it "Shirley" if it makes it easier for you. But for the sake of today's explanation, I'll call it God. Please do your best not to get hung up on the word.

God and My Ego Cohabitate in my Head

When running, I "hear" my thoughts. It's true that I have been known to speak out-loud to myself, but most of the time, I hear my thoughts in my head. But what I have noticed, is that I experience the voice of my ego, and the voice of God, slightly differently. They both live in my head, but they speak to me from different parts. Allow me to explain....

The ego lives in my forehead. I hear its voice at the front of my brain. The frontal lobe, for you nerdy types. The frontal lobe controls decision making, problem solving, control of purposeful behaviors, emotions, and consciousness. For this reason, it makes complete sense to me, that I would hear my ego voice there. After all, it's the part of my brain that believes it is me.

God lives in the back of my head, near the base of my skull. Sensations may also rise up from my midsection, heart, or throat, but they tend to form words in the back of my head, where I imagine that the spinal cord meets the cerebellum. It is a quieter voice, but it always feels peaceful and generally good. The words I hear at the base of my skull are always accompanied by a bodily sensation, often times, relaxation or relief, but sometimes excitement and joy.

I find this interesting, as the brain stem regulates unconscious functions including heart rate, breathing, and sleeping. Again, it makes sense to me that this is where I would hear the voice of God. Incidentally, the cerebellum is the part of the brain that deals with movement. If I were to imagine that God really did dwell in this part of my body, it seems fitting that I would hear His voice the loudest, while in motion.

By the way, God's voice in my head sounds just like the voice of my thoughts... the ego voice from the front of my head. The only way I can distinguish between the two is through the *place* in my body where I experience it.

If this all sounds completely nutso to you, that's ok. Frankly, it sounds more than a wee bit wacko to me too. However, it has been my experience, that when I ask a question of God, it comes from the front of my head. And when I get an answer, it comes from the back.

Talking to the Back of My Head

Once I figured this out, it made hearing the voice of God a whole lot easier. One of the things that used to happen to me before I learned that God dwelled in the back of my head, is that I would feel like I had received some sort of Divine answer to whatever question I had posed; then my ego would get to work convincing me that I made it up, that it was wishful thinking, or that I was, in fact, a total nut job. It was extremely hard for me to trust what I thought I heard. Since both voices sounded exactly the same, I felt silly and arrogant trying to discern true Guidance from ego speculation.

Now, however, the process is incredibly simple for me, and I hope that it is something that you will be willing to explore on your run today.

God's Voice and Your Happiness

One important note on happiness: It is not hearing the voice of God that promotes happiness, it's the *believing* it that matters. Happy people have faith in something greater than themselves, and they feel connected to this something. They are grateful for, and humbled by, that connection.

Today's Run

Just for shits and giggles, let's assume that God (or whatever name you give it) has a sweet little dwelling at the base of your scull too. He hangs out there, waiting for you to chat with Him, and he's a pretty awesome conversationalist. You ask questions, and he answers promptly. You can think of Him as

God, Jesus, your Ideal Self, Mother Nature, Gandolf, Professor Dumbledore, whatever... but, for today, assume that the voice of the Divine resides in the back of your head too.

As you begin your run, allow your front of mind thoughts to lead the way. They need to tire themselves out before you will be able to hear what's coming from the back of your head. So, dedicate the first ten to fifteen minutes of your run to tolerating your ego's worries, lists, grievances, and what have you. Once those thoughts have lost some of their steam, you will be ready for today's Run Yourself Happy task.

A Conversation with God

As you run, have a conversation with God. Ask Him questions, and expect to get answers. That's it. You will notice that it seems like just you, talking to yourself. But pay attention to *where* the talking comes from, and how it *feels* in your body. Go ahead and ask the Big Questions. Simply pay attention to the responses you receive.

That's it. Just notice the presence of God within you. Ask, then listen and observe.

Not receiving responses? Don't worry. Keep asking questions, and notice the thoughts and sensations that you feel immediately after. You may not "hear" God's voice, but might, instead, experience a feeling that gives you the answer. Be patient with yourself, and keep running with the intention of receiving guidance in the form of thoughts an sensations. Allow what comes without judgment. Just notice.

Post Run Journal

Write about your experience of the conversation in your head today. What happened for you?

Chapter 12

WEEK 4

Get Spiritual

Week three was some pretty powerful work, even if it felt subtle, or like you were just going through the motions. Week three can be difficult for a lot of people, as they tend to doubt themselves, or rationalize out of a perfectly good intuitive nudge. But keep it up. It will get easier the more often you practice.

This week, we will be adding a layer of spiritual practice. By now, you may have already realized that running _is_ a spiritual practice, especially when you bring the Run Yourself Happy techniques that you have learned so far, out with you on your run. This week, however, we'll be focusing on some basic elements of all spiritual practice that are absolutely essential to finding the happiness you seek.

I have no idea what your definition of "spiritual" is. Heck, I am barely coming to terms with the fact that I, indeed, *am* spiritual. So let me tell you what it means to me.

To be a spiritual person (in my eyes), means to be in touch with your Spirit. I capitalize this word, "Spirit," because I want it to feel reverent. But what is your Spirit? Well, that's the big question, now isn't it? I believe that your Spirit is that part of you that is more than your personality. Your Spirit Is. It just is. I call it lots of different things. Intuition. Ideal Self. Highest Calling. Soul. And I don' expect to be able to fully explain it adequately.

But here is what I am betting. I am betting you can *feel* it. You can feel that greater part of yourself; that wise part of your being that is connected, somehow, to the magical fabric of the Universe. There is an energy, and a wisdom, inside of you that is beyond who you understand yourself to be, and you can *feel* it.

A Story

Several years ago, I was driving home from cross country practice. I had my two year old and my three month old in the back seat, and was driving slowly down a residential street. As I drove, I got the strangest feeling that I needed to slow down, and to take my foot off the gas. This made no sense to me, as I was already driving slowly, and heading toward a green light.

I felt tired from the run I had just completed, and exhausted from being up late with the baby the night before. I remember feeling a moment of total confusion; like I couldn't stop my body from taking my foot off the gas, despite the fact that my eyes were very plainly looking at a green light. After reassuring myself, several times, that the light *was* actually green, my rational mind took over, and I put my foot back onto the gas, so that I could make the light.

Just as my front tires crossed the white line of the intersection, a car going the other direction ran a red light. I was able to slam on the brakes just in time. Had I not had that momentary, confused, battle with my body, my children and I would have been struck. My two year old would have taken the brunt of the impact. I knew, intuitively, that something greater than me had just saved her life.

Now, this was not a religious experience for me. But it was a spiritual awakening. I recognized, in that moment, that my confused, intuitive, struggle was not a coincidence. I understood, that in that moment, I had connected with a spiritual energy.

Getting Spiritual

For me, getting spiritual is simply learning how to access that part of myself, and to live more from the *feeling* place associated with it. I have found the daily Run Yourself Happy practices offered in this chapter to be immensely helpful in doing this, despite the fact that I am not a religious person. If you are religious, these may already be practices of yours, as they seem to be important components of most of the world's religions.

Gratitude. Forgiveness. Surrender.

Gratitude, forgiveness, and surrender are the Run Yourself Happy practices for this week, and they're essential tools to cultivating the whole-hearted happiness that you desire. And these three practices are undoubtedly spiritual, as they each access the loving energy that surrounds us all. Call this energy whatever you will. It has lots of names, and I tend to use them interchangeably in whatever way Spirit moves me to. But please, don't get hung up on the words. It's the *feeling* that matters. Living your happiest, full-blow miracle life, is about living from the feeling place of your Spirit. It's about living with a smile in your heart and peace in your soul. This week's practices will help to cultivate this.

As always, there are three practices suggested, but I urge you to run at least four times this week. Please continue layering the work you've done so far. I hope, by now, you are beginning to feel the shift, and that you have even begun to recognize the miracles that are undoubtedly showing up for you. This week is about going deep.

GRATITUDE RUN

Gratitude is an essential happiness practice. Notice that I didn't say that *feeling grateful* is essential to happiness. While this may also be true, it is important to recognize that gratitude, like most things, can be cultivated through practice and deliberate intention.

In her book, *Daring Greatly*, Dr. Brené Brown discusses the results of thousands of interviews with research participants. Through her work as a shame researcher, Brené Brown has discovered some key characteristics to happy people. She calls these people "Whole Hearted," which I absolutely love. Here is what she has to say about practicing gratitude:

In fact, every participant who spoke about the ability to open up to joy also talked about the importance of practicing gratitude....I was startled by the fact that research participants consistently described both joyfulness and gratitude as spiritual practices that were bound to a belief in human connectedness and a power greater than us. (p. 123)

Whole Hearted people don't just feel grateful because they have amazing lives. On the contrary. Many of Brown's research participants had lost loved ones, had businesses fail, and plenty of the other human disappointments and tragedies that we all face. These people, though, found a way to find peace in spite of these things. They chose to transcend their circumstances and find happiness, and a deliberate gratitude practice was often part of the puzzle.

Talk a New Talk

Here's the thing. If you are waiting for circumstances to change for you to feel grateful, you might be waiting forever. Unless you've been living under a rock for the past several years, it's likely that you have heard of the Law of Attraction. In case you have, indeed, been living under a rock, it boils down to this: whatever you give your attention to, and put a *feeling* energy behind, you get more of. So have a listen to yourself, will ya? Is that inner voice telling you that you don't have much to be grateful for? Or maybe you hear: "I'll be grateful when... fill in the blank." How do you feel when you think these thoughts? Sad? Longing? Less than?

Well, stop that. Stop that right now! You have the eyes to read this book. You are breathing in and out. The fact that you purchased this book means that you have enough money to do so, and the desire to get away from the discomfort of where you currently are, to a happier, peaceful, more whole hearted way of being. These are all things to be grateful for.

Get Yourself a Mantra

A mantra is simply a phrase that you repeat over and over in your head (or out loud), with the intention of focusing your attention and creating transformation. That's right, I said "creating transformation." And that's what we're aiming for, right? So try this one on for size:

"Today, I am deeply grateful."

How to Use Your Mantra on a Gratitude Run

Today's Run Yourself Happy practice is a gratitude run. I took the basic concept from one of the many Abraham-Hicks books that I have read. It is a slightly new take on what they call a "Rampage of Appreciation," and it truly works to shift your energy and put on an "attitude of gratitude." Put simply, you'll start where you are (i.e. how you are feeling), and you'll look for things to be grateful for, or to appreciate, in order to get yourself feeling better and better. You'll be using your mantra as an anchor.

As you run today, repeat the mantra, "Today, I am deeply grateful" to begin. Then, as you look around and listen to the rhythmic tapping of your feet, list the things you are grateful for. Start small, by simply noticing your surroundings, and as you run, allow yourself to be guided. Whenever you run out of things to say, simply return to the mantra. It might sound something like this:

"Today, I am deeply grateful."

"I am grateful that I am willing to try this gratitude thing."

"I am grateful that it isn't raining."

"I am grateful that my shoes comfort and support me as I run."

"I am grateful that I got myself out the door to enjoy this run."

"I am grateful for where I live."

"I am grateful for these beautiful trees."

"I am grateful for the crunch of the leaves under my feet."

"I am grateful for the trails (or sidewalks) that lead me as I run."

"Today, I am deeply grateful."

"Today, I am deeply grateful."

"I am grateful for the chirping birds, and my ability to notice and hear their songs."

"I am grateful for smiles from passerbys."

"I am grateful for my dog who loves me unconditionally."

"I am grateful for my children's smiles."

"I am grateful for my safe car."

"I am grateful that my parents are still alive and for the time I get to spend with them."

"I am grateful to be learning, growing, and expanding every day."

Today, I am deeply grateful..."

... and just keep going. Repeat yourself as often as feels right. Don't judge what comes up. Just run and repeat.

When your mind wanders...and it will, just use the mantra to re-focus your thoughts. "Today, I am deeply grateful." And be gentle with yourself. Your mind *will* wander. Just keep redirecting it back to gratitude.

The Point

The point of today's gratitude run is that you keep your mind focused on gratitude for most of the duration of your run. Whether its twenty-five minutes, or two hours, it will be time well spent.

I recommend that you dedicate at least one run a week to gratitude from this point forward. As you get more used to practicing gratitude, you may choose to dedicate a portion of each run to this mantra activity. I promise you this; as you practice gratitude, you will feel better and your vibration will shift. As you shift your vibration, you change your point of attraction, and as you do that, miracles happen!

So take your mantra with you, and spend today's run focused on practicing gratitude. You'll thank yourself.

Post Run Journal

"Today I am deeply grateful for....

FORGIVENESS MANTRA RUN

Happy people forgive.

Right now, take a minute to think about a person or situation that that you haven't forgiven. As you hold the thought of this in your mind, what do you feel?

Anger?

Resentment?

Sadness?

Disappointment?

Blame?

Betrayal?

And how do these emotions affect your ability to be happy? To be genuinely whole hearted?

You can't do it, can you? It's not possible to be fully happy while holding on to unforgiveness. And holding on to bitterness and resentment only punishes *you*, anyway, so let's practice some forgiveness, shall we?

Simple Truth:

In order to be truly happy, you must learn to forgive.

Forgiveness can be tricky business for some people to wrap their heads around. Especially, since we often refuse to forgive, because we feel wronged. I assure you that forgiveness has nothing to do with condoning wrong behavior. It has everything to do with freeing yourself. When you hold on to unforgiveness, you harbor damaging emotions in your body. If you want to release these unpleasant emotions, you must be willing to release the person or situation. If you want to experience a lighter, happier, less inhibited version of yourself, and to step boldly into your full-blown miracle life, you must begin to forgive.

The First Step is the Hardest:

Much like getting out the door for your run, with forgiveness, it's the first step that is the hardest. And the first step is, simply, to be *willing* to forgive. Once you've made yourself willing, you will be led to forgiveness. You may forgive small things at first, but once you begin to flex your forgiveness muscles, you'll use them for the heavier lifting too. So adopt an attitude of willingness. Be open to the possibility that you might someday be able to forgive, no matter how far away you think that day might be. But be clear about this: if you choose to be unwilling to forgive, you are holding yourself separate from the happy life that you desire and deserve.

You First

I've found that a simple forgiveness practice works best, and that before I can truly forgive anyone else, I must first forgive myself. Here is the mantra that I use on my forgiveness runs:

I love you, Carrie, and I lovingly forgive you.

I forgive you for…

I love you, and I forgive you for…

Then I just list the things that I am hard on myself about. I forgive myself for losing my temper with my kids, or making choices that I am not proud of. I treat myself gently, and talk to myself as though I were speaking to a sweet child. I forgive myself for being critical of my physical appearance, and being critical of others. I forgive myself for pretty much everything that feels icky, or out of alignment with love.

Usually, as I start to notice the ways in which I have been hard on myself, or the ways in which I need to forgive myself, I am reminded of the ways in which I need to forgive others. And there are a few people in my life that I must regularly forgive. These people, naturally, are the ones closest to me. I forgive my husband, parents, and children every time I do a forgiveness run. I forgive their imperfections easily, once I have acknowledged my own.

Do this

Today, as you head out the door, be willing to forgive. Use my mantra to get the conversation started in your head, but be open to letting it morph in to what it needs to be for you. Let yourself be guided simply by being willing, and start with self love.

"I love you (insert your first name), and I forgive you."

You may have to repeat this mantra for a while before it feels true to you. If you don't feel that you deserve to be forgiven, it may take several runs. But be patient. Be gentle with yourself. And just be willing. Be willing to forgive yourself and others.

Again, don't be surprised if simply repeating this mantra in your head evokes a very powerful emotional response. Just allow it, and run with tears streaming down your face, or laughing out loud. You are clearing out stuck energy and making room for more love, more joy, and more happiness. You are becoming whole hearted. Rejoice!

Post Run Journal

What was your emotional response to the run today? Write about your willingness to forgive.

GET YOUR SURRENDER ON

Happy people make gratitude and forgiveness a spiritual practice, and spiritual people make surrender a daily practice. Now, you may or may not be willing to tag yourself with the "spiritual" label just yet, but you are now three weeks into "running yourself happy," which is, undoubtedly, a spiritual practice. So, let's take it to the next level and practice surrender today.

Word Association

If the mere thought of surrender makes you uncomfortable, it is likely that the word itself is a trigger for you. It totally was for me. As a child, I learned that surrender happened in cartoons, when Wiley Coyote had finally had enough, and waved the white flag. Surrender meant defeat. And what happens when soldiers on the battlefield surrender? They are held captive by the "winning" side. In my brain, there was a huge association between the words "surrender" and "defeat."

But that's not the kind of surrender I'm talking about today. Today's surrender practice is about releasing your desires to the Universe (God, Source, etc...) in faith. And it's not defeat at all; it's freedom. It's letting go of the stranglehold of control in your life, and trusting that there is a Divine Intelligence, greater than you, that can handle the details, so that you can enjoy the ride.

So, surrender is not so much an exercise in defeat, as it is an exercise in faith. And, faith, my friends, is the game changer. Surrender is about trust. It is about knowing that there are possibilities for the manifestation of what you desire, beyond what you can currently come up with. You trust that God has your back, and you have faith that your prayers will not go unanswered.

Stop Resisting

"What you resist, persists." I first heard this saying uttered on the Oprah Winfrey show, when she interviewed several of the participants from the movie *The Secret*. What I didn't fully understand at the time was that in order to stop resisting, I had to surrender. I had to let go of my small desires to make room for the bigness of my highest calling. I had to stop thinking that I knew the way (or that I could find the answers on the internet), and have faith that a powerfully loving energy greater than me was conspiring in my favor.

That was a powerful affirmation for me: "the Universe is conspiring in my favor." And, I'll be honest; it took me years to fully understand this. But here is what I know for sure: God's got your back. And once you get that, surrender becomes a heck of a lot easier.

You simply cannot live a full-blown miracle life without surrendering to the possibility that full-blown miracles are totally possible!

What Surrender Feels Like

So, here's the thing about my surrender process: it often feels a heck of a lot like defeat, until the beautiful moment when full surrender occurs. I'm gonna go with a kind of irreverent analogy here, but I think it is one that we can all relate to. You know when you have to pee... like really bad? And you are trying to hold it, doing the potty dance, anxiously making your way to the restroom, and worried that you might not get here in time? And then you finally get there only to struggle with your pants button? But then, you finally sit on the toilet and release the flood gates. Ahhh.

And there is this moment that occurs, a few seconds after you start to pee. It's a moment of release, accompanied by a deep breath, and a feeling of total peaceful contentment. Well, that is what surrender feels like. It's like that breath of total relief on the toilet, but the relief doesn't come from the bladder, it comes from the heart. Until you surrender, you are dancing around with a very full bladder; and let's be honest, it's hard to do anything really effectively, when you have to pee.

Allow What Is

By simply *allowing what is*, we practice surrender. Awareness can be a powerful practice all in itself. Simply taking a mental step back from what we think and feel about a situation, and merely noticing that it is there. I do this with my children's behavior all of the time. Instead of getting angry and resisting their tantrums or arguments, I take a deep breath and observe. I notice that the tantrum is happening, and surrender to Love. As I do this, a miracle occurs in my perception.

In that beautiful moment, I understand that the tantrum is not showing up in my reality to piss me off, or punish me; it is there as an opportunity to open up to Love. From this place of surrendered awareness, my actions toward my children are radically different than they would be from the place of resistance. Generally, I'm able to empathize. My empathy helps my child feel understood, and the tantrum ends. The tantrum is a blessing because it is an opportunity for me to open up to love and compassion.

Take a Mental Step Back

This can be harder if your situation feels bigger than a tantrum. Perhaps you have lost a loved one. Perhaps your marriage is falling apart. Perhaps your child is sick. Or maybe your parents have wronged you. What I can offer is that there is an opportunity in every situation, to take a mental step back, observe what already is, and open up to Love and healing. Remember, miracles begin with willingness. So simply be willing to see the situation in a different light.

How to Surrender on Today's Run

Today's Run Happy practice is simple. Ask for help. Just ask God, Higher Power, Source Energy, or whatever you believe in, to help you.

"Ask, and you shall receive."

"Ask, and it is given."

So ask. Surrender to the possibility that help is available to you, and ask. What are you struggling with? Ask for help. Not sure where to start? Just try, "God, please help me. I need your help. I can't do it alone."

As you run, allow what comes up. Allow the emotions, the fears, and observe them. Just notice what you feel.

It sounds simple, but can be super powerful. Be gentle with yourself, and remember that you are bigger than your emotions. They will not break you. Surrender to what you feel in the faith that whatever shows up is here for your highest good.

Post Run Journal

What was today's practice like for you? How did it feel to ask God for help? What was your emotional response? How do you feel now?

Chapter 13
WEEK 5

Align With Purpose

My hope is that, by now, you have already felt some powerful shifts in your life. You've learned how to release stress from the body, to use the power of your imagination, to access you intuition, and have started to use your daily run as a spiritual practice. Congratulations! That is some powerful work! Take a moment to acknowledge yourself and how far you have come already.

Please continue to practice what you have already learned. This is a lifelong practice, and this book is not meant to be a quick fix, but a guide to keep you on track. This week, we'll be focusing on living your life's purpose. This can feel a bit daunting if you are still not quite sure what that is, but relax and do the work. Your purpose is speaking to you.

When You Grow Up

When you were a small child, what did you want to be when you grew up? Can you remember? If you can't remember what you wanted to be, can you remember what you liked to play?

When I was little, I wanted to grow up to be a TV star. I wanted to be onstage. But I also wanted to be a teacher. I loved playing school. I wanted to be a business owner and thought it would be the best-thing-ever to own McDonalds. And I dreamt of being a writer and a mom too (although I was pretty sure I would have six kids).

My point, here, is that when I was a child, I had more than one good idea about what I wanted to be when I grew up, but I wanted to make an impact. It is uncanny how closely those things resemble the purposeful, full-blown miracle life that I'm currently creating. I love to speak at events and through the power of online videos. I teach through my workshops and coaching programs, and I am an author, mom, and business owner. I couldn't have envisioned this exact life as a child, but it has the essence of everything I desired in a happy life when I was just a small girl.

Perhaps a better way to look at it is to notice that I had absolutely no desire to be a nurse, superhero, fireman, doctor, police officer, vet, or many other common childhood dreams. Sometimes we discount our early desires as childhood fantasies, but they're not. Your unique desires, even as a very small child, guide you toward your life's purpose.

Embracing Your Purpose

The Run Yourself Happy practices offered this week are designed to help tie the work you've done so far into the idea that your life's happiness is directly related to how genuinely you are living your soul's purpose.

For whatever reason, many people find the idea of uncovering their life's purpose to be daunting. This is usually because they don't feel worthy of it yet, or because it feels too big. I get that. I *totally* get that. And I've been there. I mean, holy crap, a few months ago, the idea of this book was just an *idea*. All I really knew of my life's purpose was that I had a fairly good inkling that I was meant to encourage, uplift, and inspire others. I knew I had a knack for helping others to develop their potential, and I knew that I wanted to do more of what I loved doing, and less of what I didn't. I loved running. I loved helping others with their lives, and I had the very best time in the world when I was able to combine the two. But that was it.

Try Not to Freak

You *do* have an incredible purpose to live out. The world *does* need your gifts, and your intuition *is* guiding you every day, attempting to steer you in the direction that your soul needs to go. But you don't need a blueprint. You don't need a ten step plan. Don't get caught up in the "how." Surrender that part to a wisdom greater than yourself. You just need have enough faith to follow the guidance that you receive.

This Week

As you run this week, you'll be revisiting some of the Run Yourself Happy practices of the previous weeks with some minor tweaks. You'll be committing random acts of kindness, revisiting your lottery win ten years later, and asking the question of "How can I serve?" Each of these activities will help you to connect to that greater part of yourself that knows exactly why you are here, and is sending you little messages and signs on a regular basis. Now that you have practiced tuning in to your intuition, it's time to flex that muscle a little more.

RANDOM ACTS OF KINDNESS

Today's run is gonna be so fun! You will be reminded that kindness and happiness are linked.

It has now been documented that even witnessing an act of kindness will raise your serotonin levels, causing you to feel happier. But, since I can't predict what you will witness on your run today, I am prompting you to actually perpetuate the acts of kindness.

At Your Core, You Are Kindness

When you deliberately cultivate kindness, you feel happier. This is because your soul *is* kindness. Being kind aligns you with your soul, which raises your vibration, which feels incredible, and attracts more kindness into your experience.

Your Assignment

Be kind on your run today. Notice who and what, are in your surroundings, and make a commitment to improve the energy that surrounds them. If you don't often encounter other people on your run, you can choose to be kind to your physical environment.

The Power of a Kind Word

Often times, on my morning run, I pass through a neighborhood full of middle school kids on their way to school. I love it when I can catch a girl standing by herself and I can complement her outfit. An unexpected compliment from a stranger is a nice way to start the school day for her, and bringing a smile to her face always feels great for me. It's an instant upper!

Being kind is also a really awesome way to connect with your intuitive, spiritual self. Be bold and trust that what you say to people is exactly what they needed to hear. If it is a kind word, it will be. Trust that you are a messenger, and say what is in your heart.

Act with Kindness

A kind act always helps me to get out of my own head and into the world around me. It's hard to have a pity party for yourself while you're helping someone else. By taking specific actions, with the intention to help or be kind, you consciously raise your own vibration and serve the world as well. It really doesn't matter how small the kind act is. The important thing is that you act.

Here Are Some Suggestions

Smile at strangers.

Stop to help someone.

Pick up trash on your run.

Pray for the people you see on the street and send them love and healing.

The mission for the day is simple: Be kind! Be kind to everyone you see on your run; be kind to the environment. Be kind to yourself as well. If you get into a lonely stretch on your run, start giving yourself compliments, or compliment your body parts. Tell your legs how great they look in your shorts, or compliment your shadow. The idea is to raise your serotonin levels.

Just Do It

So hit the streets, the trails, or wherever you run with the intention of creating your own random acts of kindness today. Be kind to your environment. Be kind to others. And be kind to yourself. Use what is available to you on your run, and create a ripple effect of good vibes in your day and in the lives of the people you encounter.

Post Run Journal

What were your acts of kindness on today's run? How did you feel before? During? After?

RE-VISIT YOUR LOTTERY LIFE

Now that you have spent several weeks going deep on your runs, it is time for a little review. Today you'll be revisiting your "Dreamrunning" Run Yourself Happy practice with a slightly different bent.

Here's the Scenario:

You won the lottery ten years ago. You bought all of the things that you wanted to buy, helped all of your struggling relatives, donated to many worthy charities, and traveled the world. You already have the life that you dreamed. So what do you do with your time these days? You're living your full-blown miracle! What does it look like? Who do you hang out with? What do you talk about? How are your days structured? What do you do to challenge yourself?

Spend the entirety of you run allowing your imagination to run free, but continuing to redirect your thought to answering these specific questions about your future reality. This Dreamrunning exercise will stretch you further than you may have allowed yourself to go before. It's important to stretch your imagination in this way for two reasons:

1. Most of the things that you think you will do when you win the lottery come from the place of believing that doing or having these things will make you happy. They

come from the false belief that you cannot be truly happy or fulfilled until you acquire them. Looking into the future, past the point of acquiring them, forces you to get to what really matters to your soul.

2. Looking at who you will be after you have achieved the miracle will point you in the direction of your life's true purpose. Because, once there is nothing left to chase, you will have no choice to listen to the call of your soul. Once you can project who you want to be, you are one step closer to becoming that person. If you are truly to live a full-blown miracle life, you have to have a clear picture of what it will be, and who you will be in it.

BONUS

And, as a bonus feature of this Run Yourself Happy practice, you will be getting yourself into the feeling place of true and lasting wealth. Which is a fabulous frequency to be vibrating from. As you vibrate out feelings of wealth and contentment, you will be attracting those very things into your reality.

Lottery Not Workin' for You?

If you are someone who struggles with the lottery idea because is simply seems too far-fetched and unrealistic, just choose something else. Whether it's a lottery win, building a business, starting a dog rescue, or traveling the world doesn't really matter. What matters is that you choose to view your life from a post-full blown miracle perspective.

Run on It

So, enjoy your run today. Connect with your future self, and feel your way into a dream existence of purpose and meaning.

Post Run Journal

Spend at least fifteen minutes detailing your post miracle reality. Be as detailed as possible, and include as much sensory language as you can.

HOW CAN I SERVE?

There is perhaps no better way to listen to your intuition or live your life's purpose than continually asking and answering this very simple question:

"How can I serve?"

As you discovered with your "Random Acts of Kindness" Run Yourself Happy practice, helping others feels good. It promotes happiness. And being of service to others is essential to living your full-blown miracle life. But today, you're going to go a little deeper. You are going to consider how you can live a life of service.

The "Sh" Word

When I first started trying to answer the question of "How can I serve?", I felt overwhelmed and anxious. I was immediately bombarded with my ego's list of "shoulds." And since we haven't talked about this dirty little word yet, I think it fitting that we address it. "Should" is a dirty word! Rebecca Shafir, author of *Zen Listening* says, "The word 'should' is probably better than any other word in the English language for creating anxiety," and I couldn't agree more. If you were to make a list of all of the things that you should do in your life, what would that list sound like? How would it feel?

My 'should' list feels like crap. Generally, our shoulds are the things that our ego has convinced us that we ought to be doing, but none of them sound like very much fun. There is good reason for this. "Should" is completely disempowering. Should makes you wrong. For instance, "I should volunteer with underprivileged children." There is an implication in this statement that because I am not currently volunteering with underprivileged children, that I am somehow wrong, a bad person, or deficient in some way. Just writing this causes me to feel guilty. But guilt, blame, fear, and other icky feelings are never true guidance. Remember that intuitive messages, inner guidance, and Divine communication always feels good in the body.

Reframe Your Should Response

As you run today and consider your answers to the question of "How can I serve?", pay attention to what comes up for you. If you get a long list of shoulds, don't freak out. That's just your ego talking. It's your mom, or the bitch in your head, or the voice of your social conditioning, but it is not your Life's Purpose speaking to you. So, here's what to do: change your "should" statements to "If I really wanted to, I could" statements.

Instead of saying "I should volunteer with underprivileged kids," you can reframe it to be "If I really wanted to, I could volunteer with underprivileged kids." From this place, you can *decide* if you really want to, or not. The thing about shoulds is that they don't really belong to us. Now, from your place of "could," you can decide if this is a way in which you want to serve. If the idea feels good, go with it.

Serve with Your Strengths

Do you know your areas of strength? Your strengths are generally things that you are good at, but you don't have to excel at something for it to be a strength. A strength is something that, while you're doing it, causes you to feel fully alive. It lights you up on the inside, and you thoroughly enjoy it. A weakness is something that, while you're doing, depletes you. You may be very good at plenty of things that are actually weaknesses for you. The trick to being of service to the world is to live in your areas of strength. This means that you do the things that cause you to feel most fully alive.

Today's Run

As you run today with the question of "How can I serve?" on your mind, pay attention only to the answers that light you up on the inside. These will likely have something to do with your areas of strength, and they may, in fact, be closely tied to some of your ambitions. That is ok. The true desires of your heart are likely tied to your Life's Purpose. Allow them to come, and don't judge them. If it feels absolutely wonderful, trust it.

Today is a good day to re-visit the "Have a Conversation with God" Run Yourself Happy practice from week three, since you will be running with a particular question in mind and seeking guidance from your highest self. And of course, practice surrender.

Post Run Journal:

Make a list of your strengths as defined above and your weaknesses. Note how many of your weaknesses are things that others tell you that you are good at. Did you get any intuitive hints about how you can serve? What were they?

PART FOUR

Chapter 14
ONWARD

Congratulations! You have run consistently for five weeks with the intention of releasing your anxiety and aligning with the call of your soul. You've used your daily run as a time to connect with your Spirit and open yourself up to your intuition. This is transformative work.

Take a moment, right now, to honor yourself. You've set your life in motion down the path it is meant to travel. Smile. Breathe that in. Feel gratitude for yourself.

You may not yet know where you are going, but it is my sincere hope that you are beginning to hear the whispers, and feel the pull of your soul. You have opened your imagination, and begun to play with raising your vibrational frequency. This is important stuff, and will absolutely make the difference between living a later version of the life you are already living, or moving into a full-blown miracle existence of purpose, fulfillment, and joy.

Stress and anxiety cannot coexist with happiness, and the only way to live a truly happy, fulfilled, and wholehearted life is to align yourself with your life's purpose and live your spiritual truth. If you are new to this work, then some of the Run Yourself Happy practices offered in this book may have been uncomfortable or frustrating for you. And that is ok.

The important thing is that you keep doing it. Just like running, the key to personal growth and development is consistency. This is why these two practices, running and personal and spiritual growth, work so beautifully together. Now that you have joined the two in your mind, you have opened a window to your soul. Your daily run is now sacred.

Moving Forward

It is my sincere intention that the practices in this book be your foundation. Running is a beautiful foundation in itself, but if you let this book be your anchor, and your intuition be your guide, I absolutely believe that you will create the miraculous life you are meant to live, one step at a time. Now that you have tried each of the practices at least once, it's time to begin again.

I offer an online program called the Run Yourself Happy System, which takes the practices in this book, and ties them into a holistic approach to finding and living your life's purpose. For more information, please visit http://runyourselfhappysystem. com. It is the perfect next step for anyone who has enjoyed this book, or needs additional support to actually implement the ideas within.

About the Author

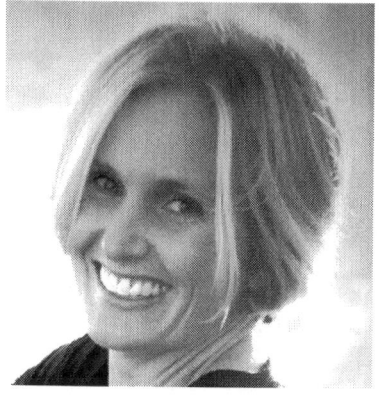

After years of sensing her own potential, but feeling unqualified, afraid, and "not enough," Carrie Roldan has stepped boldly into her purpose and has found happiness and fulfillment in the process. Carrie is the creator of the Run Yourself Happy System and an inspirational author, speaker, teacher, and coach. Carrie has three children, Quinn, Brady, and Chase, and lives in her hometown of Huntington Beach, California, where she operates a successful coaching business out of her home. Carrie has a passion for entrepreneurship, personal growth, and spiritual practice. She has found that turning her daily run into a happiness practice has completely changed the course of her life and business, and helps other women entrepreneurs to do the same. Her favorite pastime is still running and chatting about what really matters, and one of her greatest fulfillments is being able to do this with her Platinum Coaching clients.

Acknowledgements

There are so many people to thank! This book would never have been finished if it were not for the process I describe within. So my first thank you goes to the call of my soul. Thank you for your persistence. I am so glad to have connected with you.

And then, there are the people in my life who love me, and believed in me through the processes of writing, editing, and publishing. Thank to my husband Jim, and my children Quinn, Brady, and Chase.

Kareen Shackelford, thank you for being my first proof reader. Bonnie Hansen! I am so glad I sat next to you at Writing to WOW! You have been a true Godsend. And Kim Somers-Egelsee and Susie Augistin. Thank you for paving the way. Laura Jane, and Elana Arnold, thank you so much for being such inspiring and supportive friends and mentors. Emma Jeffery, thanks for telling me to stop writing that other book, and to pay attention to this one, that was whispering itself in my ear. Holly Rudnick, thank you for being my first client way back when, and showing me that what I do makes a difference. Holiday Zimmerman, and Jamie Blair-Echevarria, thanks for the years of running and chatting. You are my sister-friends, and I love you more than words can express. Thanks for simply being who you are.

Special thanks to everyone who took the time to read my book and offer praise before publishing. You'll never know the amount of confidence that gave me. Rich German, and Milana Leshinski, thanks so much for creating the Joint Venture Insider Circle. I could not have survived without this incredible community of supportive coaches. Lisa Engles, my sole sista, I'm so grateful for you and the work you are doing. I am excited to create with you.

Thank you to the team at Balboa Press and all of the kind people who held my hand through the publishing process. A big shout out to Elisabeth Diewert, who helped me to pull the trigger!

Thanks everyone who has purchased this book. You have made my dream a reality.

7909104R00099

Printed in Great Britain
by Amazon.co.uk, Ltd.,
Marston Gate.